The Seasonal Detox Diet

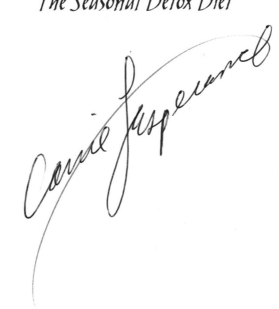

The Seasonal Detox Diet

Remedies from the Ancient Cookfire

Carrie L'Esperance

Healing Arts Press
Rochester, Vermont

Healing Arts Press
One Park Street
Rochester, Vermont 05767
www.InnerTraditions.com

Healing Arts Press is a division of Inner Traditions International

Note to the reader: This book is intended as an informational guide. The remedies, approaches,
and techniques described herein are meant to supplement, and not to be a substitute for, professional medical care or treatment. They should not be used to treat a serious ailment without
prior consultation with a qualified health care professional.

Library of Congress Cataloging-in-Publication Data

L'Esperance, Carrie, 1958–
[Ancient cookfire]
The seasonal detox diet : remedies from the ancient cookfire / Carrie L'Esperance.
p. cm.
Previously published: The ancient cookfire. Santa Fe, N.M. : Bear & Co., 1998.
Includes bibliographical references and index.
ISBN 0-89281-982-0
1. Diet therapy. 2. Fasting. 3. Rejuvenation. 4. Seasons. 5. Detoxification (Health). I. Title.
RM216 .L47 2002
615.8'54—dc21   2001051553

Printed and bound in Canada

10 9 8 7 6 5 4 3 2

This book was typeset in Berkeley Oldstyle with Kabel, Skylark, and
Rio Chico as display typefaces

THIS BOOK IS DEDICATED TO MY MOTHER, DOROTHY, AND TO
ALL OF THE ANGEL PEOPLE IN THE PAST AND PRESENT WHO
HAVE WORKED TOWARD HEALING HUMANITY, THROUGH
REVERENCE FOR EARTH AND NATURE.

CONTENTS

LIST OF RECIPES AND FASTS

Chapter 5: AUTUMN RESTORATION

Chapter 8: **HERBS**

Chapter 9: **WISDOM CHARTS**

ACKNOWLEDGMENTS

When I was a little girl, I was already acutely aware that we were taking much more from Mother Earth than we were giving back. I sincerely believe that, like the words of a favorite song, "If we give her back her diamonds, she will offer up her pearls." *The Seasonal Detox Diet* is my gift to Her. However, this book could not have come into being without the guidance, dedication, wisdom, and professional expertise of countless others who, like myself, travel the healing path.

I am grateful to the special souls who have contributed to, believed in, and encouraged the progress of this book. I am especially beholden to my mother, Dorothy, who dedicated her time to typing my handwritten manuscript over the five-year period it took to complete the work. Heartfelt thanks to Dr. Eric Suba and Michael Montgomery who contributed with their computer wizardry.

Special thanks to Barbara and Gerry Clow for inviting me to be a part of the Bear & Company publishing family; to editors John Nelson and Sonya Moore for helping to make the text "sing." My background in film and photography has helped me appreciate the talented people who have helped create the design elements for *The Seasonal Detox Diet*. Generous thanks to text designer Melinda Belter. I gratefully acknowledge Chef John Ash for all of his contributions to this work.

In the year this edition was published the winds of change blew in and Bear and Company was sold to Inner Traditions. I gratefully acknowledge and thank all of the dedicated people at Inner Traditions/Healing Arts Press for their enthusiasm, artistry, and fine-tuning skills in preparing this book for its second printing.

Thank you to Rob Meadows for contributing his thoughtful and patient marketing expertise during the difficult decision to change the title from *The Ancient Cookfire* to *The Seasonal Detox Diet,* and to Peri Champine for the lovely new cover she designed. My project editor, Janet Jesso, did a great job in getting all the bugs out of the text right down to the bibliography. Thank you, Janet!

A final thank you to each reader who sees the wisdom in *The Seasonal Detox Diet* and profits from its treasures to progress along the healing path now, and always.

Be Well

SPECIAL NOTE TO READER

In regard to health- and healing-oriented information, this book is to be considered as a reference work. As such it is intended solely for use as a source of general information and not for application to any individual case. The material draws from time-honored healing systems as well as the author's own personal experience. It should be noted, however, that the opinions expressed herein are not necessarily those of, nor endorsed by, the publisher; nor can the publisher certify that use of the procedures, recommendations, or substances contained herein is safe or will produce the results described in each individual case.

The information contained in the following pages is in no way to be considered as a substitute for consultation, diagnosis, or treatment by a duly licensed physician or other health care professional. Such professionals are in a position to evaluate each individual case and suggest appropriate measures, depending on the circumstances.

INTRODUCTION

WHAT WE THINK AND WHAT WE EAT
MAKE WHAT WE ARE,
PHYSICALLY AND MENTALLY.[1] [288-038]

—EDGAR CAYCE

True knowledge of healing ways is scattered everywhere, like pieces of a gigantic puzzle. A great wealth of information has accumulated over thousands of years, from the past into the present time, within the many cultures of the world. Each piece of the puzzle represents many journeys and many teachers, each offering a unique way of helping to form the healing picture. When consolidated, these works become a potent, valuable, and holistic application more relevant than ever in today's society.

The Seasonal Detox Diet contains an invaluable array of dietary wisdom and culinary art collected by this writer. It is based on research over a span of twenty-five years of studying the best health and dietary systems the world has to offer, from before the time of Hippocrates to the present. There is much to learn from long-forgotten historical experience as well as today's scientific inquiry. Given the knowledge, we can strike a balance between the modern world and the ancient; utilizing the old as well as the new is not a paradoxical situation. The ancient truths are as valid and real today as they were yesterday, and modern science has shed more light on them.

We have all traveled to many cookfires—from the crackle and glow of an evening campfire as we prepare our meal, to the aromatic cup of tea in Chinatown or even to the city street vendor's wagon of roasting chestnuts on a crisp winter morning. These are meeting places that entice us with the promise of a nurturing experience. It is not only the nourishing food and drink, but the uplifting of our senses and spirits, too.

The ancient cookfire was the central place where people gathered to rest, keep warm and dry, prepare their foods, eat, and socialize. The tasks of meal preparation and the sharing of food assisted greatly in creating a fertile environment for the spoken story. Depending on the attitude with which we listened, we might obtain guidance and gain knowledge and wisdom through conversations of the day. Whether you wandered in as a known acquaintance, or you were lost or maybe an adventure-seeking traveler, the cookfire was and still is a place of nourishment for our bodies, minds, and spirits.

Thousands of years ago, people in the Far East realized that not only body structure but even human nature can be changed by attending to the manner in which we eat and drink. For these ancients, eating and drinking were considered the most important rituals in the divine art of life. Among other cultures, culinary art is also an art of life: The Sufis, for instance, hold that our health, happiness, liberty, and judgment are all affected by what happens in our kitchens.

Today, according to the U.S. Surgeon General, many conditions are dramatically improved, even cured, with correction of diet and lifestyle. Clearly our physical, psychological—even spiritual—well-being depends largely upon what we eat, how it is cooked, and the way we eat it. As the brilliant natural systems designer Bill Mollison wrote in his book, *Permaculture,* "people are built up molecule by molecule, cycling through themselves the materials of their environment: its air, soils, foods, minerals, and pathogens. Over time, people create their own ecology. Any system or organism can accept only that quantity of a resource which can be used productively. Any resource input beyond that point throws the system or organism into disorder; oversupply of a resource is a form of chronic pollution."[2]

There is the story of a wise old Native American woman who, when asked by her visitors how they could help heal Earth, replied, "Heal yourself." The concept seems simple, yet it is a strange one to many. It is a challenge we all face. Recognizing responsibility for our own health, we then care for others by caring for ourselves. We help heal our earthly home by healing ourselves. The possibilities are infinite.

The Seasonal Detox Diet makes it easy to explore these many techniques that have been, and still are, essential for health and self-healing. They are all tried and tested to help ensure a pleasant and rewarding time. The book is designed to take you on a healing journey that will cover restorative cleansing diets and special fasts essential for achieving balance physically, mentally, and spiritually. Chapters include history, research, philosophies, concepts, and recipes to help you in the restoration process of your body.

Once you incorporate these healing practices into your life, it is easy for your body to rebuild itself through what you eat and how it is prepared; you will find an eclectic blend of simple and more exotic dishes especially chosen to facilitate the natural healing processes of the body throughout the seasons. These recipes maximize the use of the best ingredients available, from the much-loved Kumari Curry Dressing for vegetables and greens to Pumpkin Custard Pie. They are all carefully crafted to complement the principles in the culinary art of life and healing that unfold throughout this book of knowledge and wisdom.

I became fascinated with nutrition at a very young age, due to my own physical difficulties, and learned that health is not something you can take for granted or that necessarily comes easily. I had to work at informing myself. My curiosity initiated a lifetime study of world healing systems from Ayurveda to folk medicine, including esoteric vision-ary Edgar Cayce's as well as Native American healing systems. The common thread of these systems is that they all use food and fasting in basic therapies to treat illness and to maintain health. Therapies involving food and fasting are known as preventive medicine, or self-healing, if you will—a do-it-yourself maintenance program.

In traditional Chinese medicine, the doctor's role is to help patients learn how to take care of themselves. Teaching the patient is as important in the long run as prescribing an herb or drug. The physician is also thought of as a gardener. The human body is consid-ered a garden where each species is connected to every other. The physician's task is to tend the garden the way you tend roses—to cultivate and nourish. The physician should teach patients to be gardeners, too, and help them understand how to summon the heal-ing faculties of their own bodies for recovery. In old China, the doctors were only paid to keep people well; when their patients became ill, the doctors had to take care of them free of charge. An effective insurance policy indeed!

We do not have to become fanatics in order to reap the rewards of good health. People do not have to sacrifice the pleasure in their lives for it. But we may have to sacrifice some of the super-busyness of life, the frantic and wasteful activities that we all go through every day. We have let the increasing busyness of modern life crowd out the thoughtfulness that can make being busy more fruitful. In folk medicine we hear that our emotions are some-how involved in our physical well-being. Now science, too, is telling us that there is, in fact, a relationship between our emotions and our bodies—that emotions can have both adverse and positive effects on our immune system for example. In a sense, healing is not about medicine but about an attitude toward living and caring for ourselves and for each other. It is a philosophical quest, not just a scientific quest.

We are at a turning point, where it is time to reexamine and rethink our meals, kitchens, cookbooks, grocery stores, and land use—as well as food waste and energy waste—in relation to health care and policy. At this time, government health programs, health care costs, and toxic medicines from pharmaceutical companies are troubling our nation. Our wisest choice is to educate ourselves regarding our own bodies and to look to the simplicity of Nature for our health. Nature embodies mysteries that modern technol-ogy has not yet fathomed. The study of natural healing takes a lifetime, and there is always something new to learn.

The accumulated skills, customs, styles, ideas, and wisdom from the people of history have become readily available. Among these are tools with sacred value. As we enlarge our awareness of our world heritage from all societies, we add to the meaning of our own experience. In *The Tibetan Book of Living and Dying*, Sogyal Rinpoche states that "all the spiritual teachers of humanity have told us the same thing, that the purpose of life on Earth is to achieve union with our fundamental, enlightened nature. Undertake the spiritual journey with all the ardor and intelligence, courage and resolve for transformation that we can muster. There is the path of wisdom and the path of ignorance. In this time of violence and disintegration, spiritual vision is not an elitist luxury but vital to our survival. To follow the path of wisdom has never been more urgent or more difficult."[3]

The purpose of this book is to consolidate and present the wholeness of understanding required to keep our living art (our bodies) together. We are the creators of our own health, and we have to utilize all the resources available to create healthy bodies, minds, and spirits. This process is more important than we can even grasp as a whole. As George Ohsawa, the Japanese macrobiotic nutritionist explains, "you must heal yourself before attending to anything else."

The Seasonal Detox Diet

REAL "FASTING" DOES NOT ENTAIL GIVING UP EATING AND DRINKING ENTIRELY.
FASTING MEANS ABANDONMENT OF THE HABIT OF GREED WHICH CAUSES US
ALWAYS TO EAT AND DRINK IN EXCESS; FASTING IN THE TRUE SENSE MEANS TO
EAT AND DRINK "SIMPLY" IN ACCORD WITH THOSE PRINCIPLES WHICH ARE AT
THE CORE OF THE INFINITE ORDER OF THE UNIVERSE. FASTING, TOO, IS AN
ANTIDOTE TO OVEREATING.

—GEORGE OHSAWA

CHAPTER ONE

RESTORATION

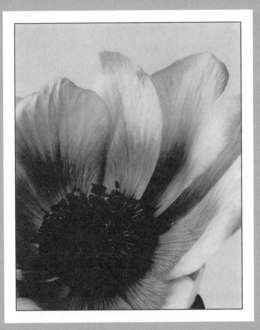

RESTORATION (RES-TO-RA'SHUN) N: THE ACT
OF RESTORING; RENEWAL; REPAIR. TO BRING
BACK TO ITS FORMER STRENGTH; REBUILD;
HEAL OR CURE; AMEND; RECLAIM. A FOOD
OR MEDICINE HAVING THE POWER TO
RESTORE.

RESTORATION

Among the many pearls of wisdom in natural healing is this statement: "Illness can be the doorway to health." Whether the illness originates in the mind, body, spirit, or environment, we have the choice to allow illness to compel us either toward health and higher learning, or away from health and to eventual destruction.

It is not surprising that about 50 percent of people in the United States now use alternative therapies, both to maintain health and to treat illness. However, alternative therapies are, in truth, not so alternative. Many of them have actually been utilized for thousands of years. Many people in this country are using them as important additions to Western allopathic medicine. The evidence is overwhelming that people who take care of themselves have lower health care costs.

Preventive medicine in particular is a kind of health insurance that pays interest. Preventive therapies require that people take part by achieving awareness and body conscious behavior by actively participating in and being responsible for their own health. Preventive therapies enable us to feel confident that what we do now to avoid medical bills will help us overcome or deal with future health care crises. We are looking toward our later years, a time when life should be fruitful and satisfying.

The beauty of eating seasonal foods and using cleansing diets is their simplicity and their ability to help balance the systems of the human body. Most anyone can achieve noticeable results in a very short time! Though the methods are simple, there is still much to learn. The many recipes offered here are treasured for their effective healing abilities, and all involve some type of food and drink.

Food is vital because it is the primary source of gaining energy. Everything around us has its own unique kind of energy or vibration. Some foods increase energy more than others. Depending on the way they are grown, prepared, and eaten, foods have the ability to increase or decrease the vitality and the strength of body, mind, and spirit. This fundamental knowledge of foods has always been with us.

Today the quality of our earthly environment has a net effect on physical health. Commercial kitchens, supermarkets, agribusinesses, and systems of food distribution are industrialized and immensely complicated. Radiation, food additives, genetically engineered foods, and overprocessing are just a few of the problems we deal with today. Our bodily elimination systems were not designed to decompose substances totally foreign to us. Pesticides, decayed matter, food additives, dead protein, certain inorganic minerals, and a number of other substances simply do not belong in our bodies. The condition of our bodies also reflects the condition of our environment, our world, and our future on planet Earth.

We can be overwhelmed by toxic accumulations as a consequence of fatigue, poor circulation, constipation, drugs, alcohol, tobacco, improper diet, and our environment. As the body becomes increasingly toxic, proper oxidation cannot take place in the tissues. Without oxygenation, we lack energy so the tired body continues the downward spiral. Restoring our own bodily systems after years of constant wear is essential for maintaining health and preventing disease. This creative process empowers us to become responsible for our own health and teaches us to care for this fascinating human body in its relation to Nature and the four seasons.

Clarissa Pinkola Estés describes the body as a sensor: "Many times it is the things of nature that are most healing, especially the very accessible and the very simple ones. The body is like an Earth. It is a land unto itself. It is as vulnerable to overbuilding, being carved into pieces, cut off, overmined, and shorn of its power as any landscape. We tend to think of the body as this 'other' that does its thing without us. Many people treat their bodies as if the body were a slave. We have only to pay heed to our bodies to know what we must do. The body is not sculpture or marble. Its purpose is to protect, contain, support, and fire the spirit and soul within it, to be a repository for memory, to fill us with feeling. It is to lift us and propel us, to prove that we exist, that we are here, to give us grounding, heft, weight. The body is best understood as a being in its own right, one who loves us, depends on us, one to whom we are sometimes mother, and who sometimes is mother to us." [1]

The importance of being "mother" to my body hit home when I was in my late twenties. During many years of studying nutrition, I felt I had taken care of myself with good eating habits. Imagine my alarm and confusion upon realizing my health was deteriorating a little more with each passing year. Constant allergies made it impossible to be anywhere without a box of tissues. I began to have night sweats and insomnia. Seasonal colds and flus came and lingered long. It did not seem to matter how much care I took with my diet. It was at this time, while reading Dr. Walker's book *Raw Vegetable Juices,* that one small paragraph about detoxification caused a lightbulb to go on in my head—and I have never looked back. The message was simple: "Cleanliness is the first step toward a healthy body." [2] This was an important but missing link for me: We can regenerate the body when clean tissues are able to draw all the nutrients and chemical elements we need from the foods we eat. We cannot put clean food in a dirty body and expect good results. Accumulation and retention of waste and morbid matter in our bodies begins in the womb and continues throughout childhood and up to the present moment. We are not necessarily what we eat; we are what we are able to assimilate, digest, and utilize. If the organs of our bodies are clogged and congested, we cannot expect to function optimally—and we do not!

About 2,500 years ago, Hippocrates is said to have offered the Grecian people wise advise: A healthy mind in a healthy body should be the goal of all generations in the world. Hippocrates was a vitalist who taught that good health and purity of environment are dependent upon each other. Over time, pollutants build up in the tissues of our inner environment and cause our bodies to fall out of balance and weaken. Various forms of disease are then able to take hold when the body is in this weakened state. Many others since the time of Hippocrates have known that the body comes back into balance with the assistance of correct diet.

Hippocrates was an enlightened physician; his first step in maintaining health was regimen, or a regulated mode of life. He knew that Nature made the cure and that the doctor's role was to assist. He believed that the diseased body needed a period of rest—not only a physical rest, but a chemical rest, which he considered even more important. Chemical rest could be achieved only by withholding food, thus giving the organs of the body an opportunity to discharge accumulated waste products and thereby to cleanse themselves.

We go about the restorative process by the use of special cleansing and dietary fasts. Fasting is the oldest form of natural healing. Many authentic world healing systems, which include Ayurvedic, Unani Tibb, Chinese, Japanese, Sufi, Native American, and European folk medicines, utilize herbs, foods, and fasting to achieve balance and health. Internal cleansing is the foundation of preventive medicine. Utilizing food and fasting to heal the body offers the benefit of helping the body to detoxify itself from the variety of pollutants evident in our modern environment. Many people intuitively sense the need for this detoxification.

The principle of fasting is based on the basic structures and processes of the human body, mind, and spirit. Some people confuse fasting with starvation and find various ways to talk themselves out of this healthful practice. The sense of hunger often disappears in people who completely abstain from food—both those fasting and those starving—but the similarity ends there. The process of fasting is one of gradually aligning more and more with the body. It is actually the epitome of a natural way of life, and its benefits do not end with correcting our out-of-balance systems and restoring our health.

"Restoring balance physically and mentally through right diet and fasting can change the individual human constitution, the intellectual tendency, the sexual inclinations, and social behavior slowly and steadily in the direction of total health,"[3] explains Japanese nutritionist George Ohsawa. The great visionary Edgar Cayce proclaimed: "The body physical is truly the temple through which the mental and the spiritual and soul development must manifest, and in manifestation does the growth come."[4] [5439-1]

The methods of fasting employed throughout history range from discontinuance of a single food for a short time up through total abstinence from all foods and liquids for extended periods. In the present day, fasts must be adjusted to suit the times. These all involve certain combinations of food and drink. If you are reasonably well, most fasts will bring about an almost euphoric feeling of well-being and provide inexpensive and effective insurance against disease. If you are not well, the fast is an excellent beginning of a therapeutic program.

The corrections the body makes can be subtle or powerful. Hering's Law of Cure states: "All cure starts from within out, from the head down and in the reverse order as the symptoms first appeared."[5] The law of cure for healing the body moves symptoms from inside to outside, from top to bottom, from more important organs to less important organs. The movement may stir up your most recent symptoms of disease, or it may reawaken your oldest ones. Old problems may reappear for a short time, but they will fade. It will not take long for peaceful healing signs to emerge, and these signs will let you know you are doing a good thing for yourself.

The Sufis probably have more experience performing fasts than any other group. They point out that natural symptoms or "healing crises" are precisely the events that Western medicine labels illness and disease. Many people are unwilling to endure any discomfort or unpleasantness whatsoever when ill and thus resort to various chemical drugs, which will unfortunately put an immediate end to any healing actions of the body. This may suffice to get a person back to work, or prop him or her up to attend an important function; but over years of suppressed eliminations, the toxic matters back up within the system until organ damage occurs and there is no hope for a cure, except by the most drastic measures. (The physical manifestation of illness may also be the effect of a deeper problem involving your emotional and mental body. When you address the cause, your body must follow suit.)

While fasting the severity of the symptoms in a healing crisis is usually related to the amount of stored toxins in the body. You may experience headaches, cold or flu symptoms, constipation, depression, skin eruptions, or fatigue. In many cases, the possible effects the detoxification triggers are much less dramatic than you might imagine. In most cases, these symptoms are a good sign that you are allowing your body to heal itself. However, your medical history should be taken into consideration. If you feel concerned about any symptom, you may wish to call your physician. Some people go through cleansing fasts with few symptoms.

A cleansing fast will encourage the body to release stored toxins from muscles, glands, tissues, and fat cells into the bloodstream for elimination through the lungs, kidneys, intestines, skin, and the menstrual cycles for women. If elimination is impaired, these toxins cannot be eliminated quickly enough, which creates some of the uncomfortable symptoms. To help relieve this toxic burden, the internal baths are very important. You will learn much about your own needs as you progress through your fast. It is important to observe and utilize disturbances as stepping-stones for higher, better, and greater understanding of your body's needs. Remember to be patient while fasting, knowing that healing must arise from constructive thinking and application on your part.

When the body is cleansed, the eyes sparkle, the skin becomes soft and clear, the mind is sharp, and the manner is calm and pleasant. Everything gets better, including the memory, circulation, and digestion. These benefits are only the beginning. Health and happiness can become as contagious as disease. If we work on our health only when we are ill, we will usually return to the place where we started. Or, we can work on our growing health and not become ill. The willpower and discipline for proper care of nourishment, exercise, and self-awareness are not easy, but then nothing of value ever is.

Fasting has been likened to a surgeon's knife: It does away with toxins of all kinds. We must ask ourselves what is wrong with us, and then direct the fast to the purpose in the correct manner. In chapters 3 through 6, you will find time-proven therapies for healing used in many parts of the world and administered in the clinics of famous physicians. Many of these practices are very simple, refreshing, and delightful. Others are more time-consuming and regimented. It is important to choose wisely and become comfortable with your self-therapies.

THE ART OF FASTING

People who are not familiar with fasting may imagine that it entails sitting around getting bored and depressed, and not eating anything. Some of us are even convinced we will die if we miss a meal. At times it is difficult to slow down the pace of life enough to even think about giving the body a break. The more disconnected we are from our bodies, the more difficult it is to imagine the powerful effects that fasts using certain food and drink can have. It is quite an adventure in itself and fascinating to learn about the body, mind, and spirit by challenging yourself in this way.

There is much you can do to keep you busy during a fast. There are schedules to keep, special combinations of food and drink to be prepared, and a host of other enjoyable treatments such as various baths, skin brushings, and massages. You may wish to take advantage of special therapies by health practitioners. It is important to acquaint yourself with the many methods and recipes developed throughout history for fasting. These methods create the "work" of fasting; it is up to you to decide how intricate the work will become, depending on personal resources.

Fasting reduces fat in the body. Women enjoy a firm waistline and men are delighted when the "love handles" or the "spare tire" around their waists disappear as a benefit of fasting. The body becomes less congested and is able to reshape, restore, and retexturize itself once the purification process begins. Of course, this does not always happen instantaneously; for most of us it occurs gently and consistently through correct diet over time. In his most recent studies, Dr. Bernard Jensen often tells his patients not to expect a full recovery in less than a year. In our lives we need a sense of constant renewal. This exhilarating feeling of renewal is consistently achieved with restorative fasting diets. Each time I have fasted, my body has indicated when to start and when to stop, and I have found this to be true in fasting experiences of others as well. Each time you fast, you will learn something new about yourself and the hidden gifts with which self-healing will reward you. Do not let your health take a backseat to anything. You are your own best guardian.

It should be noted that some people have a tendency to go overboard. In their excitement and effort toward restoring the body, they reason that if a little does this much good, a lot more may achieve even better results. This kind of thinking can create more harm than good. The methods given are time-tested and proven, so please follow the instructions as directed to achieve the "best" possible results—no more, no less. Once you become familiar with fasting and the effect it has upon your system, you will naturally be able to make adjustments in the recipes to better suit your own needs.

EXERCISE AND FASTING

Exercise should be kept to a minimum while fasting; this is a time for the body to do work internally. Walking and light gardening are good physical activities to assist metabolism during your fasting experience. Simple yoga exercises that are not too strenuous will help to balance and stimulate your inner organs during a fast. It is important to develop and maintain a regular exercise pattern after completing your fast. The body needs exercise to ensure proper nutrient absorption. Exercise also triggers the well-known "feel good" hormones in your system, the endorphins, which are the morphinelike opiates of the brain that calm and reassure. They are responsible for giving a lift to the spirit and increasing metabolism.

WHO SHOULD ABSTAIN FROM FASTING

Those people in very weakened states, such as cancer patients, should not undertake cleansing fasts. Pregnant women and very young children also should abstain from fasting. The alcohol- or drug-dependent person should seek individual treatment and consultation while fasting from a carefully chosen professional in the field of natural medicine. If you have diabetes, heart disease, ulcerative colitis, or epilepsy; if you are not yet age eighteen, or are more than 10 pounds underweight; if you are on medication, you need special supervision while fasting. If you have any questions about fasting, whatever your medical condition, please consult a naturopathic physician. See Sources for referrals.

In general, you should not lose a lot of weight while fasting unless you do an extended water fast—which is not recommended in this book. Fifty years ago, a fast on water alone was advocated as safe and effective—not so today. Most people have accumulated DDT— among other dangerous pesticides—in their fatty tissues. A water fast loosens these foreign accumulations, but instead of being directed through the liver into the large intestine to be eliminated, they are driven into the bone marrow. This is the last place we want poisons to accumulate. For this reason, a cleansing fast on water alone is not advisable or recommended.

OBSTACLES

I am referring now to dependence on smoking, drinking, or drugs. There are so many health risks related to overindulgence or dependence upon these detrimental practices that I cannot recommend them to anyone, particularly while fasting. In most cases, cleansing the body of accumulated toxins will relieve the craving for nicotine, alcohol, and other drugs.

Those who avoid cleansing the body because of these addictions are the ones who are often in "greatest need" of fasting to achieve balance. The body does have the ability to constantly renew itself if given a chance. Therefore, regardless of what habits govern us, we need only to possess the genuine desire—along with sincere determination and willpower—to become balanced in body, mind, and spirit.

If you smoke and are addicted to nicotine, do not allow it to deter you from taking a step forward regarding your health. Cut down as much as possible while fasting. If the urge to smoke becomes overwhelming, chew on a piece of licorice bark, swab a tiny bit of clove oil onto the back of the throat, or try smoking herbs such as damiana leaves (calming) and rosemary (menthol taste). As an aid in quitting tobacco, try smoking lobelia, also known as Indian tobacco. It contains lobeline, which is similar to nicotine but does not have the same addictive effects. There are a number of commercial herbal cigarettes available that are also useful in making the transition from smoking to stopping.

If you are recovering from alcohol dependency, certain herbs are good to include in your diet. They can also be used while fasting. In China and Japan, the kuzu root has been used by herbal doctors as an anti-alcohol herb for thousands of years. It is valued for its actions on reducing alcohol consumption by neutralizing acidity and thus relieving minor aches and pains. Highly nutritious kuzu root starch is used in much the same way as arrowroot, cornstarch, gelatin, or flour to thicken sauces, stews, and puddings; it also makes vitalizing teas. Kuzu root powder is much higher in calcium, vitamins, and minerals than any other ingredient used for thickener. It is excellent in teas and soups for colds, flus, and digestive and intestinal disturbances of many kinds. Kuzu is a valuable super-food to add to the diet. Its use in the future as a nutritional supplement for alcohol-dependent people looks promising. In 1993 researchers at Harvard University Medical School and the University of North Carolina Bio-Medical Research Laboratory began studies on the mild actions of this valuable plant. Kuzu root starch is available at your natural foods store and should find a permanent place in your cooking.

❁ KUZU REVITALIZING TEA

Dissolve the kuzu root starch in the cold water, add the gingerroot, and heat until the tea begins to boil; stir the tea until thickened. Remove from heat and blend in the tamari and umeboshi plum. Drink $1/2$ to 1 cup from 1 to 3 times a day as desired for nutritional support.

INGREDIENTS	AMOUNT
kuzu root starch	1 heaping tsp.
pure water (cold)	1 C.
fresh gingerroot (grated)	$1/10$ tsp.
tamari	$1/4$ tsp.
umeboshi plum (minced) (optional)	$1/2$ tsp.

Medicinal-strength herbal teas (see chapter 8 for recipes) that are excellent for aiding those suffering from the effects of alcohol include: angelica, elecampane, goldenseal, hops, maize, mullein, parsley, plantain, red clover, sage, wormwood, and yellow dock. These herbs also help to calm, cleanse, strengthen, and nourish the ailing tissues of the body. For more information see Sources.

The long-term toxic effects of drug residues from many drugs, including marijuana, cocaine, and LSD, can be modified by detoxification. Many of these drugs are stored in fatty tissues, as are industrial chemicals and pesticides. People with "historical" residues will be amazed at the clarity of mind they experience as they purge their bodies of contaminants and street drugs.

Drug-depleted brain and body chemistry can be restored using amino acids and other nutrients therapeutically during early recovery. More than a thousand programs nationwide have begun using nutritional therapy for dramatic improvement in moods and reductions in cravings. Look for therapists who are licensed by your state to practice this particular nutrient therapy.

IF YOU ARE UNABLE TO COMPLETE YOUR FAST

If you need to end your fast before it is completed, it is very important to break it slowly by drinking juices and broths and eating only raw or steamed vegetables and fruits for at least the first day or two. Consuming a large or difficult-to-digest meal, such as cooked meats, will shock your body out of its cleansing state and may cause discomfort or illness. You will feel the benefit of your fasting effort and your body will adjust accordingly, continuing to build on this process, if you maintain a diet that consists of at least 75 percent vegetables and fruits. Do not expect all of your energy to return immediately after you stop fasting. It takes a few days to build full strength; then as time passes, you will discover that you are stronger than ever.

CHAPTER TWO

THE FOUR SACRED SEASONS

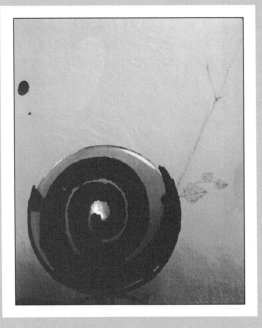

WHEN SPEAKING OF ONE DAY,
THE MORNING IS GOVERNED BY
SPRING,
AFTERNOON BY SUMMER,
EVENING BY FALL,
AND NIGHT BY WINTER.
THE SPRING ENERGY GIVES BIRTH,
THE SUMMER PRODUCES MATURITY,
THE FALL IS THE TIME FOR GATHERING IN,
AND THE WINTER IS A TIME FOR
STORAGE.

—NEI CHING[1]

Time, privacy, and peace are the perfect combination during a fasting experience. If you find it difficult to achieve all of the above, do not allow it to dampen your enthusiasm. Challenge yourself to be creative. Each of us must find our comfort zones through trial and error. My mother did her first cleansing fast while working as a secretary, and she reported increased energy and elation throughout her 10-day fast. On the other hand, by the third day of my first two fasting experiences, I contracted a terrible headache that lasted through the night. I knew these were toxins being released and suffered through it. I felt weaker through the duration of a 6-day fast, but enjoyed a strong spiritual clarity and balance never before experienced. The first 24 hours of a fast can be the most difficult regarding the craving for solid food because the body is accustomed to being fed every day and is expecting to expend the large amount of energy it takes to digest each meal. Once the body attunes itself to this regimen, a new metabolism kicks in and directs the surplus energy to cleansing and purifying; the special foods help accelerate and assist the cleansing process.

If you wake up one morning and decide that the time is ripe to harvest the new you, by all means be spontaneous about it! As you integrate the idea of fasting into your lifestyle and begin to understand the processes of your body blueprint, you may decide to plan your fasting days to coordinate with the magic of the seasons, or special times of the week, month, or year. Seasonal restorative fasting attunes us with the cycles of Nature. Fasting can be a dedication or a ritual with special significance, purpose, and meaning or a cleansing experience to help your body overcome colds or flus.

Ask yourself what you want to achieve, then begin in full acceptance of your inner self. This is a good time to take a vacation from anything stressful, if possible. Some fasts are easily utilized while in working situations; others may require a more restful time for the body to heal. Very inexpensive fasts can be planned throughout the cycles of the planting and harvesting seasons when you or your neighbors may have an abundance of fruits and vegetables on hand from gardens. These make excellent juices and foods for many basic cleansing recipes.

BODY SYSTEMS AND NATURE

The four sacred seasons mark definite power releases on Earth. During the four-day interval introducing each of these seasons, the currents of desire are largely stilled so the spiritual forces can predominate. You can learn much from observing the cycles of Nature and the daily motion of the Sun and Moon. Times of seasonal change are important as reorganizational periods, for increasing self-awareness and looking at life priorities. Seasonal changes are also times of greater stress and thus of potential illness or physical difficulty. Your adaptability to these changes is vitally important to your continuing good health.

The two equinoxes and the two solstices are the high points of the natural year. All of Nature comes into attunement with spiritual energies released at these times. Each individual act and manifestation of creativity arises from a mysterious ground of inspiration and is mediated into form by a translating and communicating energy. Artists, writers, poets, musicians, and other creative workers often merge themselves with the inspiration to be found at this time; their creations are often endowed with an outpouring of the same energies.

The solstices and equinoxes are traditional benchmarks in understanding the cyclical nature of time that has been passed on by the world's most ancient civilizations. The Maya, who occupied the lowland areas of coastal Belize as early as 1200 B.C., possessed a deep awareness of humankind's place in the cosmic scheme of things and the sacredness of all creation. The ancient Maya constructed ceremonial centers, temples, and pyramids aligned with the heavens. When viewed from the top of these pyramids, the sun rises directly over the middle temple on March 21, the spring equinox; from behind the left-hand temple on June 21, the summer solstice; over the middle temple again on September 23, the autumn equinox; and from behind the right temple on December 21, the winter solstice.

Powerful leaders of nations, of religions, and of societies sometimes make a point of abstaining from food for several days at a time to clarify their thinking, to increase their willpower, and to become better people; Mahatma Gandhi is an example. In the book *Staying Healthy with the Seasons*, Dr. Elson M. Haas explains that Oriental healers learned that, in each season, two interrelated organs get stimulated to cleanse and rebuild. Food choices can either block this natural cleansing cycle or help it to flow.[2] It is wise to fast during the change in seasons because the body adjusts the fluids as the seasons change. A fast during these times will help you to move smoothly into this transitional period, void of illness. We will utilize the Chinese system of the Five Element Theory (Wood, Fire, Water, Earth, Metal), which also correlates with the Native American healing systems, to assist in understanding the relationship of the various body systems in association with Nature.

SPRING EQUINOX

Spring is one of the most important times to cleanse the body. The beginning of spring, March 21, is the time of the spring equinox, when day hours equal night hours. For the next 6 months, the sun will be dominating our lives.

The spring season is correlated with the element Wood, which governs the gallbladder and liver, important filtering systems for the blood. These are the organs of the body to which a fast may be directed for spring cleansing. Diets for the liver and gallbladder are offered in chapter 3. Even if you choose not to do a restorative spring fast, Springtide Fare offers delightful maintenance recipes featuring foods to help the body move smoothly into spring and stimulate cleansing.

SUMMER SOLSTICE

We enter summer on June 21 with the summer solstice, when the Sun is at its northernmost position relative to Earth. At the solstice, we have the longest daylight of the year, but it also marks the beginning of the cycle of growing darkness. Summer is Nature's season of growth and maturation. Flowers, fruits, and vegetables are all around us and our gardens abound with fresh, live foods for cleansing and restoring the body.

Fire is the element characterizing summer; it is seen to provide the energy governing the heart and small intestine. The heart, one of the organs most active in the summer season, is the regulator of blood circulation. Pay attention to it in summer, along with the small intestine, which absorbs most of the nutrients for the body from the foods we eat. To care for the heart and small intestine, consult chapter 4. Summertide Fare follows Summer Restoration with special recipes highlighting great summer foods that help maintain, restore, and cleanse your body in the season of the sun.

Late summer is regarded as a transitional season. The restorative cleansing diets offered at the end of chapter 4 focus on the stomach and the spleen. Transitional recipes are also included. Earth is the element correlated to this time.

AUTUMN EQUINOX

Autumn is one of the most important times to cleanse the body. The autumn equinox begins September 23 in the Northern Hemisphere; it is the time of the Sun's passage south across the equator. Autumn marks the beginning of a cycle of personal turning within; its first day is the equinox day, when night's darkness again is equal to the length of day. The days of seasonal change around the autumn equinox are a perfect time to cleanse your body and lighten yourself for fall's work. Like early spring, early autumn is a good time for cleansing, but afterward your diet may be fuller, richer, and more heat-producing than in spring, in order to carry you through the chill of late autumn and winter.

The element Metal is associated with autumn; it represents the mineral ores and salts of Earth. The lungs and the large intestine are the two organs that get stimulated to cleanse at this time. The autumn season is a good time to work at keeping these organs strong and healthy. If you have a history of digestive or bowel weakness, or of long winter colds and lung problems, this is the time to prepare yourself for staying well this fall and winter with the excellent cleansing diets for the large intestine and lungs found in chapter 5. At the end of the chapter, Autumntide Fare recipes enrich the palate with fall foods to strengthen and protect you in this season of breathtaking colors, acorns, and crisp autumn weather.

WINTER SOLSTICE

Winter is the most difficult time for fasting. Great care should be taken in choosing winter foods to build strength and to guard against illness. The winter solstice begins on December 21 and reaches its climax of spiritual power at midnight on December 24 when, it is said, jubilant hosts chant the midnight birth of a new sun. Mother Nature is hibernating, silent; the roots prepare for spring. December 21, the first day of winter, is the time of the longest night. Daylight increases gradually after the winter solstice.

Winter is related to the element Water. The bladder and kidneys, which deal with the body's water, are the organs associated with this element and this season. Water is the essential medium of your body through which all things pass. This fluid of life is necessary for functions such as circulation of the blood, elimination, and lymphatic flow. Beneficial cleansing diets and recipes for winter are offered in chapter 6.

SACRED HOLIDAYS

Incorporating fasting into your lifestyle will increase your sensitivity and enhance your intuition. In the book *Shakti Woman,* Vicki Noble emphasizes the importance of being aware and open during specific times of the year. "There is a deep, underlying psychic structure that the ancient people knew about and worked with in their daily lives that has been lost for the most part in the present day. What geomancers have called dragon lines and what English dowsers call ley lines are part of a grid system that surrounds our planet: crisscrossing lines along which energy and force pass in regular paths that can be felt and, to some extent, harnessed by people. Ancient megalithic builders (like those who built Stonehenge) knew about this grid and built structures on important points of power or current. The ancients used knowledge of the grid system for observing their seasonal festivals at certain precise times delineated by the movements of planets and stars in relation to Earth. There is evidence to support the belief that the earliest of builders on Earth observed these particular points on the calendar."[3]

These sacred holidays are universal in their meaning. They date from the most ancient times and recur throughout history in many lands; they even show up in our secular calendar today. If we look more closely, the derivation of the two major Christian holidays becomes apparent: Winter solstice became Christmas in the Julian calendar and Easter follows the spring equinox. The four essential sacred days that fall between the solstices and equinoxes, called cross-quarter days, go relatively unnoticed in Western culture. They usually are considered "children's holidays" such as May Basket Day—or May Day—and Halloween. Yet these cross-quarter days hold the most power astronomically and are celebrated by other cultures around the world as sacred days belonging to the Goddess (the deep feminine).

Celtic peoples celebrated these holidays with bonfires until the most recent times. The Swiss national independence day falls on August 1, the eve of Lammas (August 2), the high point between the summer solstice and autumn equinox. There remain many remnants of these ancient practices of our ancestors, who worshiped these cycles with reverence and devotion. Even the groundhog, looking for its shadow on February 2 —Candlemas—the high point between winter solstice and spring equinox, is a reminder of the oracular powers available at that time and of the prophecies that were once made in the name of Brigit.

It is not necessary to do anything in particular to celebrate the sacred days. The main thing is the power of the moment. These holidays are part of an undergirding structure of forces and currents that affect us in all kinds of ways and that move and guide us spiritually, whether we know it or not. The intensity rises at these times of the year, and it is said the door opens between the visible and invisible planes. People respond to this by becoming upset, angry, euphoric, energized, or sick. What is needed, once you know about the timing, is to prepare a space for your own reception of the energies that are available. Give yourself time to dream and remember, allow some space for reflection and observation. Stay awake! Whatever happens in your life at these particular times is oracular—it tells or shows you something. It presents you with messages, signs, and omens about your life. "Big" dreams are likely to occur then, as well as other unusual psychic events. Synchronistic and magical happenings are possible. We in the West often get hung up on "doing something" for the holidays, when the real goal is to let the holidays "do" us.

ANCIENT WHEEL OF SACRED HOLIDAYS

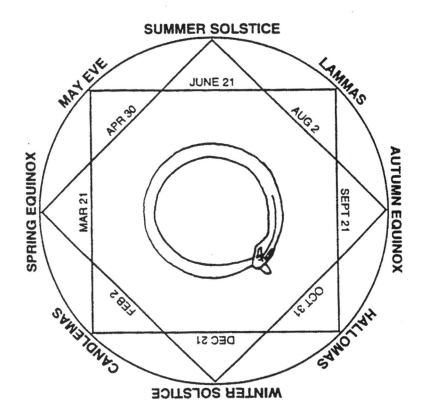

SUMMER SOLSTICE

MAY EVE

LAMMAS

JUNE 21

APR 30

AUG 2

SPRING EQUINOX

AUTUMN EQUINOX

MAR 21

SEPT 21

FEB 2

OCT 31

CANDLEMAS

HALLOMAS

DEC 21

WINTER SOLSTICE

IF YOU DESIRE GREATER SPIRITUAL FULFILLMENT YOU MIGHT ASK YOURSELF, "AM I TAKING GOOD CARE OF MYSELF IN EVERYDAY LIFE?" BALANCE BEGINS TO BE RESTORED WHEN WE STOP TAPPING INTO OTHERS FOR OUR ENERGETIC CHARGE, AND LOOK INSIDE OURSELVES FOR OUR CONNECTION TO SPIRIT.[1]

—JAMES REDFIELD

CHAPTER THREE

SPRING

RESTORATION

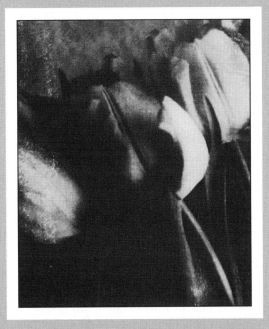

BUT FOR LIFE THE UNIVERSE WERE NOTHING; AND
ALL THAT HAS LIFE REQUIRES NOURISHMENT.[2]
—*FANNIE MERRITT FARMER*

SPRING CLEANING

The spring season is a very important and inspiring time to do a cleansing fast. Our bodies begin to respond to the changing season by releasing foreign matter or toxins and mucus. By supporting our bodies with cleansing foods during this process, we can accomplish very deep cleaning and come much closer to achieving optimum health. After a long winter of eating heavy foods, it is refreshing to cleanse and lighten our systems as we see the tender buds and blossoms emerge in this season of renewal. If you are fasting for the first time, it is a good idea to choose a simple recipe such as the Spring Equinox Fast, the Lemonade Diet, or Fasting on Apples, until you become more familiar with how your body will react.

In traditional Chinese and Native American healing systems, the **liver** and the **gallbladder** are the two interrelated organs that get stimulated and should be cleansed in spring. If you want to keep your liver and gallbladder in good condition, a varied range of fasts is offered here, from the simple to the more detailed and time-consuming. The tender spring-green dandelion is valued for its restorative effects on the liver and gallbladder. Though it is beneficial to do any fast in spring, this is indeed the best time to cleanse the liver and the gallbladder. These organs perform essential body functions, particularly the digestion and processing of many substances we take into our bodies. Take a moment to familiarize yourself with this chapter before you embark upon your fasting journey.

🌹 SPRING EQUINOX FAST

All of the fruits and vegetables needed to stimulate the body to cleanse and eliminate in spring are contained in this simple fast based on the Chinese Five Element Theory. Choose the foods that are readily available in your area from the list below. Natural foods markets often stock fresh dandelion leaves along with fresh parsley. These are good spring herbs to add in small quantities to fresh apple or vegetable juices. The foods in this fast can be eaten in either solid or liquid form, so this is an easy fast. A 3-day fast helps the body get rid of toxins. A 5-day fast starts the healing process. A 10-day fast completely cleanses and renews your bloodstream. A 10-day fast is beneficial twice annually—once in spring and once in autumn. I like to clear the digestive tract with the Epsom Salts Internal Bath given in chapter 7 before starting this special diet; you may omit this step if you prefer. Skin brushing (p. 198) each day is also recommended.

TIME: Spring
TIME FRAME: 3 to 10 days

8 A.M. to 12 noon: kiwis, oranges, limes, grapefruit, lemons, apples, applesauce (unsweetened), apple juice; pure water and herbal teas.

The above foods can be taken in solid or liquid form. Choose one or more and eat and drink as much as you like until noon.

12 noon to 8 P.M.: asparagus, beets, broccoli, cabbage, carrots, cauliflower, dandelion leaves, garlic, leafy greens, olive oil, parsley, parsnips, potatoes with skins, sprouts; pure water and herbal teas.

The above foods can be taken in solid or liquid form. The vegetables can be raw, steamed, baked, or roasted, and a simple dressing can be made from the olive oil, garlic, and parsley. It is best to have a combination of raw and cooked foods at each meal to supply the live enzymes needed for proper digestion.

❀ GALLSTONE CLEANSE

If you wish to cleanse your gallbladder follow the above diet with the addition of drinking one quart of fresh-pressed apple juice per day. The malic acid in the apple juice will soften the stones. The malic acid, however, is present mainly at the skin of the apple. On the sixth day skip dinner and at 6 P.M. take 1 teaspoon of Epsom salts dissolved in warm water and citrus juice. Repeat at 8 P.M. At 10 P.M. make a cocktail of 4 ounces olive oil and 4 ounces fresh squeezed hot lemon juice. Shake vigorously and drink. Go to bed and lie on your right side for 30 minutes. In the morning you will pass green stones varying from the size of grains of sand to some as large as your thumbnail. You won't feel a thing, and depending on the shape of your gallbladder you may be amazed!

MENU TO BREAK THE FAST

Build on this diet by adding spring grains such as barley, quinoa, wheat, millet, and rye. Eat plain yogurt flavored with vanilla extract and spices, goat's milk cheeses, and free-range chicken, turkey, or fish once a week if desired. (Refer to acid-alkaline section in chapter 9 to balance your diet healthfully.)

❧ EDGAR CAYCE'S APPLE DIET
TIME: Spring
TIME FRAME: 3 days

The apple is eaten whole in this fast adapted from the *Edgar Cayce Handbook for Health*.[3] It is very simple and excellent for cleansing the whole system in general. The apple diet is very energizing; it is amazing how good it makes you feel. Organic red and yellow apples may be used. Yellow apples contain the most pectin, a substance that helps to reduce cholesterol.

This cleansing diet may be repeated once a month for 2 or 3 months. It is a purifying diet to clear the whole alimentary canal, the liver, kidneys, and your system in general. Recommended apple varieties include Jonathan, Jenneting, Black Arkansas, Oregon Red, Sheepnose, Delicious, and Arkansas Russet.

For 3 days eat nothing but apples. You may drink coffee if you desire, but do not put milk or cream in it, especially while you are taking the apples. Drink plenty of pure water. On the morning of the fourth day, take about 2 tablespoons of olive oil.

❧ THE LEMONADE DIET

This diet is adapted from the Master Cleanser recipe developed in the United States by Stanley Burroughs. It is a simple cleanse that also sustains energy enough for even heavy working situations. Lemon and lime are perfect liver foods and great body

INGREDIENTS	AMOUNT
pure water (warm or cool)	1 C.
fresh lemon or lime juice	2 T.
cayenne pepper	to taste
maple syrup	1 or 2 T.

cleansers. High in vitamin C, potassium, and other minerals, they are somewhat astringent—they contract and tighten tissues—which loosens and clears the toxins from deep tissues and organs. The cayenne pepper helps to clear the blood and eliminate toxins and mucus as well as keeping the body warm. The maple syrup offers energy and is delicious and full of minerals.

This method dissolves and eliminates all types of fatty tissue at the rate of about 2 pounds a day for most people, without harmful side effects. In all diseases such as the flu, asthma, hay fever, sinus problems, bronchial troubles, and colds mucus is rapidly dissolved and eliminated from the body, leaving you free from various allergies that cause difficult breathing and clogging of the sinus cavities. Cholesterol deposits in the arteries and veins also respond to the magic cleansing power of the lemonade diet. Skin disorders may also disappear as the rest of the body is cleansed.

PURPOSE
- To dissolve congestion in any part of your body.
- To cleanse the kidneys and the digestive system.
- To purify the glands and cells throughout your body.
- To eliminate waste and hardened material in joints and muscles.
- To relieve pressure and irritation in the nerves, arteries, and blood vessels.
- To build a healthy bloodstream.
- To keep youth and elasticity of tissues regardless of your years.

The lemonade diet is recommended for a minimum of 10 days; it has all the nutrition needed during this time. Note that the use of honey or any other sweetener is not an acceptable substitute for maple syrup.

Drink the lemonade as needed when hungry or thirsty throughout the day; a minimum of 6 cups should be taken. The ingredients can be adjusted to suit your taste. No solid foods are eaten, but it is important to keep the intestines moving daily to clear toxins. Any of the internal and external baths (chapter 7) are excellent additions to juice fasting.

MENU TO BREAK THE FAST
DAYS 1 AND 2: 8-ounce servings of fresh orange juice as desired during the day to prepare the digestive system to assimilate other foods. May be diluted with water.
DAY 3: Orange juice in the morning. Raw fruit for lunch. Fruit or raw vegetable salad at night. You are now ready to eat normally.

❧ HERBAL TEA FOR SPRING FASTING

One cup of sassafras tea daily for a few weeks during spring will help cleanse the whole system. It is known to purify the blood and cleanse the kidneys, bladder, stomach, lungs, skin, and joints. Used both internally and externally, it has been helpful in easing poison oak and poison ivy itching, as well as rheumatism and arthritis. Sassafras has an enjoyable flavor; it should be used in small amounts.

INGREDIENTS	AMOUNT
sassafras bark	1 tsp.
pure water	5 C.
whole clove buds	5
fresh vanilla bean	1 inch
kuchica twig or pau d'arco	1 T.
peppermint	1 T.
horsetail	1 T.

In a glass or stainless-steel saucepan, simmer the first 5 ingredients for 10 to 15 minutes. Remove from heat and add the peppermint and horsetail. Cover tightly and allow to steep for 15 to 20 minutes longer. Strain and enjoy.

THE LIVER

The liver is the body's largest internal organ. This master laboratory is located in the right upper abdomen. It conforms to the under surface of the diaphragm (the breathing muscle that separates the chest from the abdomen). The lower liver edge can often be felt under the rib cage on the right side of the body. Essentially, it stores and distributes nourishment for the entire body, is involved in the formation and breakdown of blood, and filters toxins (unusable materials) from the blood.

The ancients respected the liver and believed it to be not only the soul's center but the most important organ in the body. It is a tough gland, able to rebuild itself and function with less than one-fifth of its whole. The blood supply of the liver is almost entirely venous—the most impure blood, carrying the waste of the body. The liver is the body's principal organ of detoxification, the strainer through which pour all the impurities that find their way into the body before entering the general circulation.

Overeating can lead to an enlarged, overworked liver. Too much of any food, but especially alcohol, chemicals, drugs, fried foods, and meats, can be toxic to the liver and gallbladder. From the natural viewpoint, when the liver is overloaded, it is less able to detoxify the blood, so poisons remain. When it becomes impaired, the toxins enter the circulation and cause irritation, destruction, and eventually death. That is why you must guard your liver so carefully. The liver is one of the organs greatly afflicted in this time and age. Keep this organ in the best possible shape with a spring fast for the liver and gallbladder, yearly or biennially.

STANDARD LIVER FUNCTION TEST

The primary circulation of blood through the liver is via the portal vein; when there is liver congestion, a back pressure of blood into the whole venous system occurs. The increased vein pressure can easily be detected by the following simple test: With your fingertips, press down on the skin. Lift your fingers. If a blanched, white area remains, it is an indication that increased vein pressure, or plethora, exists. When the vein pressure is normal, no white area is noticeable. This test may be made on the skin of the chest, inner legs, or back and will give the same result.

LIVER FLUSH DRINK

It is well known that alcohol will overburden the liver. If you should "overdo it" by having too much to drink, the next morning help your liver with this special drink, a prescription of Dr. Randolph Stone, father of Polarity Therapy.[4]

INGREDIENTS	AMOUNT
fresh lemons	*1 or 2*
olive oil (cold-pressed)	*1 T.*
garlic or small piece of gingerroot	*2 cloves*
pure water	*1/4 C.*

Squeeze the lemons and add the remaining ingredients to the juice in a blender. Blend 30 seconds and drink. After drinking this mixture, relax or exercise for a bit, then drink a cup of warm fennel, anise, or fenugreek seed tea.

SEED TEA

Simmer ingredients for 15 minutes in a covered stainless-steel or glass pot. Let tea sit for another 15 minutes, strain, and drink.

INGREDIENTS	AMOUNT
fennel, anise, or fenugreek seed	*2 tsp.*
pure water	*2 C.*

This tea assists the action of the liver flush and also acts as a relaxant and carminative (relieves gas) in the digestive system. After a half hour, eat a light breakfast of oranges to help balance the overacidity the alcohol creates in the system.

LIVER AND PANCREAS STIMULANT

This drink stimulates pancreatic digestive enzymes to help restore and rebuild the liver. Pancreatic enzymes are essential for fat and protein digestion.

INGREDIENTS	AMOUNT
pure water	*1 C.*
nutmeg	*1/2 tsp.*
vanilla extract (optional)	*1 or 2 drops*

Warm the water and steep the nutmeg in it for 5 to 10 minutes. Add vanilla. This drink can be made with cool water if desired. Take as a morning beverage or 1/2 hour before meals.

THE GALLBLADDER

The gallbladder, a saclike organ, sits behind the liver. It stores and secretes bile for digestion, especially for the breakdown of fats. Improper gallbladder function may cause gas
and cramping in the abdomen, most commonly in the right upper abdomen, as well as
"referred" pains to the shoulders and the back between the shoulder blades. Congestion
of the gallbladder energy may manifest itself in physical and mental tension, especially in
the shoulders and head, but also in the hips and thighs—areas connected with the gallbladder's energy pathway. Headaches, both tension and migraine types, are related to the
gallbladder in the Chinese system.

Gallstones are formations of crystals of cholesterol or, sometimes, bile salts. The stones
may be as small as grains of sand or as large as walnuts. A gallstone attack occurs when a
stone becomes wedged in the duct that carries bile from the gallbladder to the intestines.
However, many people with gallstones do not experience symptoms. A gallstone attack
can be triggered by a meal laden with hydrogenated fats and hard-to-digest fatty foods.
These include foods made with overheated, often rancid, oils: french fries, potato chips,
popcorn, and donuts. When symptoms occur, there may be sudden pain in the upper
right side of the abdomen that lasts for several hours after a meal. Fever, chills, and vomiting may also occur. Most often, a gallbladder attack resolves itself as the stone passes.
However, if the stone is lodged in the common duct serving both the liver and gallbladder, blocking all bile flow, jaundice and possible liver damage may occur.

The following liver and gallbladder spring fasts are useful for keeping the gallbladder
free of stones.

AMISH REMEDIES FOR THE GALLBLADDER

To keep the gallbladder in good shape and to encourage cleansing during spring, these
time-tested Amish folk remedies are valued.

🌹 REMEDY #1

Warm 1/2 cup pure water and dissolve 1 tablespoon Epsom salts in the water,
stirring until clear. Add an additional 1/2 cup cool water; set aside. Juice 3
lemons and blend in 1 tablespoon cream of tartar (see note below). Combine
the lemon and water mixtures and keep in a cool place. Take 1 tablespoon of
this solution each morning before breakfast (until it is finished). Keep your diet
simple—mostly dark green vegetable salads with cold-pressed olive oil dressings
and apple juice. Avoid fatty foods and meats.

Note: After grapes have been fermented in wine making, the deposits or lees at the bottom of the cask or barrel are refined to make one of the main ingredients in baking powder. Avoid cream of tartar if you are allergic to sulfites.

 REMEDY #2

Upon arising, take 1 tablespoon fresh parsley juice with 1 tablespoon pure water. Eat a diet of fresh greens with cold-pressed olive oil dressings and apple juice or apples. Before retiring at night, drink the juice of 1 or 2 fresh lemons, undiluted, then lie on your right side for 20 minutes. This is good to practice for 2 to 4 days.

 REMEDY #3

Take 1 teaspoon cold-pressed olive oil, followed directly by 1 teaspoon fresh lemon juice. Do this morning, noon, and night, while fasting for 3 consecutive days on fresh green vegetable and apple juice combinations, adding an equal or lesser amount of pure water. For best results, use the internal bath of your choice while fasting.

AMISH REMEDIES FOR GALLSTONES

 REMEDY #1

To soften gallstones and clear them from the gallbladder, eat nothing but grapefruit or drink only fresh grapefruit juice until relieved of the stones. Uva ursi tea (p. 154) should accompany this fast. *Note:* Avoid citrus if you have stomach ulcers.

 REMEDY #2

Before retiring, take 6 ounces pure cold-pressed olive oil with a bit of warm water or lemon juice. First thing in the morning, take 1 teaspoon Epsom salts dissolved in warm water, stirring until clear. Keep the diet simple and focus on fresh citrus and greens until relieved of gallstones. *Note:* Avoid citrus if you have stomach ulcers.

DANDELION FOR SPRING CLEANING

Dandelion, "the tooth of the lion," is a good springtime healer. Whether the dandelion is a native of North America or a naturalized plant is debated by authorities; either way it is found and eaten in most parts of the world. All parts of the dandelion are used, either for food or medicinal purposes—the leaves and crowns for salads and cooked greens, the flowers for making wine, and the juice for warts and blisters.

The dandelion root is a blood and kidney cleanser and tonic, as well as a diuretic. It can be used as a general cleansing stimulant for the liver. Both the dried leaves and the dried and powdered root are used as a bitter tea. This tea is for any malfunction of the liver. Fresh dandelion leaves or dried root are valuable additions to a diet for people with diabetes and hepatitis. (Check with your naturopathic physician before taking any herbal remedies for such illnesses.)

The main benefit of this great herb is to enhance the function of the liver, but the root is also useful for clearing obstructions of the spleen, pancreas, gallbladder, bladder, and kidneys. It is of tremendous benefit to the stomach and intestines, balancing the enzymes that simultaneously benefit digestion, assimilation, and elimination. Dandelion root helps lower high blood pressure, thus aiding the action of the heart, and it can also be helpful in treating anemia by supplying necessary nutritive minerals. If you have always thought of dandelions as weeds, perhaps now you can see them as edible tonics and digestive aids, and as stimulants for cleansing the body.

I use the herb dandelion in the following fast for the liver and gallbladder. This is a detailed version of this special fast. If you prefer a simple example of this cleanse, try the Simple Gallbladder Flush on page 34.

✿ LIVER AND GALLBLADDER FLUSH
TIME: Spring
TIME FRAME: 3 to 4 days

This special fast based on European folk medicine will cleanse and revive both the liver and the gallbladder whenever needed. The ideal time to begin is 3 or 4 days before the spring equinox, when hunger is at an ebb due to the approaching equinox. This elaborate version is designed to achieve optimal results in helping to restore the liver and to flush stones from the gallbladder. Unless the diet has been excellent throughout one's lifetime, there are few of us who would not benefit from cleansing these organs. Prepare for your fast a day or two ahead of time by gathering the ingredients you will need. During this time, eat simple light foods such as fruit, vegetables, and grain dishes that move through the system easily. Take an herbal laxative tea before going to bed the night before you begin. I like to use Epsom salts or castor oil and drink mainly juices, broths, and herbal teas the day before the fast to cleanse and empty my digestive tract in preparation for the fast. Instructions for internal baths are in chapter 7.

The following recipes contain the main foods used. The time frame for fasting on the juices should be 2 to 4 days, depending on how long you feel you should fast. If you are over age forty, a longer fast may be needed to break up gallstones.

Note: Skin brushing is a very beneficial way to stimulate your inner organs. Fasting is a perfect time to introduce your body to this important healing "bath." It takes little effort, only a few minutes of your time, and is a good habit to adopt, especially while fasting. Do it each day before dressing or showering. Skin brushing is explained on page 198.

❁ WARM APPLE JUICE

Prepare 1 quart at a time as needed. Apple juice should be organically grown, fresh-pressed juice or cider, brown in color—not the clear type

INGREDIENTS	AMOUNT
apple juice	*4 C.*
cinnamon sticks (whole)	*2 or 3*

or canned variety. The pectin and malic acid in fresh-pressed juice made with unpeeled apples are what soften gallstones.

Gently warm the apple juice and cinnamon sticks, being careful not to heat it to boiling. Remove it from the heat. Cover tightly and allow to steep 20 minutes before using. This is the main juice you will drink throughout the fast. Fruit juices are cooling to the system, and the addition of cinnamon balances the juice with a warm metabolic heat for digestion and delicious flavor. If cinnamon is unacceptable to your palate, try 2 or 3 whole cloves or some nutmeg, or just drink plain apple juice. Fresh-pressed apple juice will keep well for a week or two refrigerated, and it freezes well, remaining delicious and healthful even when slightly fermented. This juice is also combined with the following dandelion herbal tea to cleanse the liver.

❁ DANDELION HERBAL TEA

Simmer the dandelion root in the water, uncovered, for 20 minutes, then strain the liquid over the dandelion leaf. Cover tightly and steep for another 20 minutes; strain the tea again. Keep this tea separate from the apple juice, only combining the two when called for during the fast.

INGREDIENTS	AMOUNT
pure water	*4 C.*
dried dandelion root	*6 T.*
(1 year old minimum)	
dried dandelion leaf	*6 T.*
(double amount if fresh)	

BASIC TIME SCHEDULE FOR FAST

DAYS 1 THROUGH 4: Solid foods are not eaten at all during the first 2 days of this fast. Instead, 2 different drinks are taken 2 hours apart for a total of 7 times each day. The drinks are cleansing and nutritional; they should be thought of as food. The first phase of digestion begins in the mouth, so savor the flavor, slowly. "Chewing" a beverage mixes it with saliva, which is what happens with solid food.

8 A.M.: $1/2$ cup each warm apple juice and dandelion tea, combined.

10 A.M.: 2 cups plain apple juice plus $1/2$ cup water.

12 noon: 1 cup each warm apple juice and dandelion tea, combined.

2 P.M.: 2 cups plain apple juice, $1/2$ cup water, $1/2$ cup fresh-pressed beet juice, combined.

4 P.M.: 2 cups plain apple juice plus $1/2$ cup water.

6 P.M.: 1 cup each warm apple juice and dandelion tea, combined.

8 P.M.: 2 cups plain apple juice.

Follow this schedule for a minimum of 2 days or a maximum of 4 days. Any of the internal and external baths (chapter 7) are an excellent addition to this fast. The coffee and vinegar internal bath (p. 189) is recommended particularly for deep liver cleansing.

At the end of your fast, about 3 hours before your bedtime, the most challenging part of this fast will be at hand. It is not as hard as it sounds, and it is much less trouble than going into the hospital for a gallbladder operation.

First, lay a doubled 12-inch square of cotton or wool flannel on a plastic bag and carefully soak the fabric with castor oil. You will also need a warm heating pad or hot water bottle. To open the gallbladder ducts in preparation for the olive oil cocktail, take $1/4$ teaspoon Epsom salts dissolved in $1/3$ cup warm water. Chew on organic orange or lemon rind if the taste of the salts is disagreeable. Wait 15 minutes, then take the following cleansing drink.

❧ OLIVE OIL COCKTAIL

Use a blender or wire whisk to mix the ingredients. Drink this down with a little more hot apple-lemon juice if needed.

Get into bed and lie on your right

INGREDIENTS	AMOUNT
cold-pressed olive oil	$1/3$ C.
cream	$1/4$ C.
apple juice (hot)	$1/3$ C.
fresh lemon (juice only)	$1/2$ or 1 T.

side. Place the castor oil pack on your liver and gallbladder area—just below your ribs on your right side. (Cover with plastic, a small towel, and the heating pad.) Apply the heat for 1½ to 2 hours. Remove the pack. Then take the Epsom salts mixture a second time—in the same proportions—and begin to drink fresh citrus juices slowly. Cleanse the skin, if needed, with a mild solution of baking soda and warm water. You should rest easily, but if you have difficulty with nausea, oranges relieve this sensation; chew the orange well, and do not eat too much of it. This fast is based on diets practiced in health spas and hospitals in Europe and the United States.

In general, this fast starts to work by the next morning. It cleanses the liver and gallbladder tract of old bile and debris such as gallstones. The old stagnant bile becomes dissolved and liquefied by the malic acid of the apple juice, and the oil drink moves it out. In your eliminations, you may find various-sized pebbles that range from bright green in color to muddy brown. These are gallstones formed by rancid fats in the diet.

A colonic irrigation or enema on the day after completion of this fast is excellent to encourage rapid release of toxins. In an individual more than forty, it may take several fasts for the gallstones to break loose.

MENU TO BREAK THE FAST
To help heal the liver and gallbladder after your fast, avoid all fried foods, heated oils, and fats. Fried foods create bad cholesterol for the body and are best avoided entirely throughout one's lifetime. Especially avoid heated oils that are combined with starches such as french fries, potato chips, baked goods, and breaded fried foods. The foods listed in this menu should be eaten in 8- to 10-ounce servings.

BREAKFAST: 1 or 2 fresh whole oranges, pineapple, grapefruit, or berries; herbal tea (choose from liver/gallbladder herbs).

MIDMORNING: Fresh-pressed apple-beet or carrot-beet juice with celery.

LUNCH: Small salad of your choice, concentrating particularly on green leafy vegetables, cucumber, watercress, celery, parsley, and fresh herbs. Combine fresh plain yogurt with the Kumari Curry Dressing (p. 42) for a delicious salad dressing treat.

DINNER: Fresh soups, salads, steamed vegetable dishes, or whole grain breads, rice, or millet (choose one starch).

This is a good general menu to stick to for several days after completion of your fast. Avoid overeating at all meals and keep in mind that drinking liquids during a meal of solid food dilutes the digestive acids in your stomach and inhibits digestive action in the whole body. Build and strengthen the organs with the liver and gallbladder herbal combinations listed on the following page.

❧ SIMPLE GALLBLADDER FLUSH
This is the simplified version of the Liver and Gallbladder Flush. Fast for 24 to 48 hours on organic raw apple juice. Cleanse the colon each day with the coffee and vinegar internal bath (chapter 7). Before bedtime on the last day of your fast, combine ½ cup olive oil with ⅓ cup hot apple, lemon, or grapefruit juice and drink. Lie on your right side for ½ hour before going to sleep. In the morning, you should pass the softened stones. After your fast, build and strengthen the liver and gallbladder with the foods and herbs given. Use the herbs in teas and capsules as additions to a sensible daily diet.

LIVER AND GALLBLADDER HERBAL COMBINATIONS
When the liver and gallbladder are unhealthy, herbs and herbal combinations should be used to cleanse and nourish, increase circulation, feed the nerves, and harmonize the whole system. These herbal combinations offered by Louise Tenney also benefit the kidneys, pancreas, spleen, and age spots.[5] Use the Standard Medicinal Tea recipe on page 213 to prepare these herbal tea combinations.

❧ HERBS FOR COMBINING #1
Red beet, dandelion, parsley, horsetail, liverwort, black cohosh, birch, blessed thistle, angelica, chamomile, gentian, and goldenseal.

❧ HERBS FOR COMBINING #2
Barberry, ginger, cramp bark, fennel seed, peppermint, wild yam, and catnip.

ALOE VERA JUICE
Aloe vera juice mixed with papaya puree is my favorite drink to stimulate digestion and sooth the entire digestive tract after completing any fast. Aloe vera offers so many benefits that it should find a place in your fasting experience or everyday diet regardless of the season. In Sanskrit, aloe is called *Kumari*, which means "Goddess"; it is used each day by East Indian women to maintain beauty and counteract symptoms of aging. In the West, aloe

vera gel is considered one of the most effective healing agents for the treatment of burns or other skin injuries. A diluted aloe vera liquid can be taken daily for its enzyme-promoting activity.

Aloe vera figures prominently in gynecology. Ayurvedic medicine considers aloe gel to be estrogenic, which accounts for its vitalizing and tonic properties for women. Taken daily for at least 3 months, a teaspoon at a time or in combination with turmeric root, aloe regulates liver function, balances the female hormones, and counteracts symptoms of pre-menstrual syndrome.

Native to Africa, aloe vera has been naturalized in most of the tropical zones, but in North America it grows only as a house plant. The aloe vera plant is invaluable for its magical ability to heal many internal and external irritations—from rashes, stings, and sores to constipation, ulcers, and colitis. The plant's excellent reputation dates back as far as 1700 B.C., when aloe vera was highly respected as an "all purpose" remedy—an antibiotic, astringent, complexion smoother, skin healer, stomach mender, and pain reducer. When broken, the long, succulent leaves exude a thick gel that is very soothing and healing to burns and minor cuts. The gel from a broken leaf may be rubbed on the skin as a beauty treatment; it nourishes the skin and prevents and diminishes wrinkles.

Internally, aloe vera is excellent for aiding the digestive organs and has a very soothing effect. When used in the diet, it also has the ability to kill any unwelcome bacteria in the intestinal tract. However, once these are eradicated, the overuse of aloe vera can also begin to destroy the beneficial bacteria. Few herbal plants need to be constantly used in the diet—aloe vera is one best used for 3 months on, 3 months off, throughout the year.

❀ ALOE-PAPAYA JUICE

Combine equal parts of aloe vera juice with papaya puree concentrate to create a delicious drink that will sooth the stomach lining and stimulate the whole digestive process very effectively. Aloe vera and papaya in combination make one of the best and most delicious drinks to indulge in after completing any fast. The digestion is noticeably improved in a very short time.

To make aloe vera juice, simply cut open the green leaf of the plant and remove the gel with a spoon. Liquefy the gel in a blender, or soak it in water under refrigeration for a few days, then liquefy. Use 2 to 4 ounces of aloe vera juice mixed with your favorite juice or ginger tea. Dry the green leaf and store it for 1 year; the leaf can then be used as a laxative for your fasts.

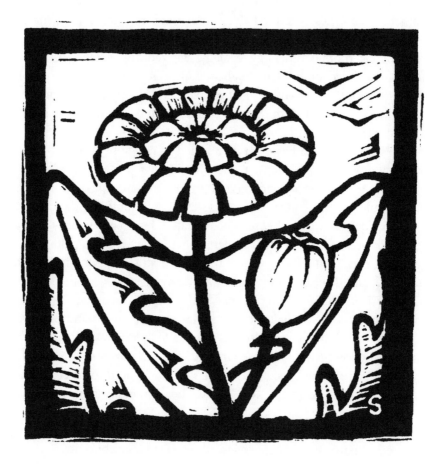

Nature provides no written test on her laws. She only smiles or frowns faintly on her subjects, and whispers softly in approval or disapproval of their conduct. Her disciplines seem very mild, even to the most careful observer, but in the long run, continued obedience to her laws leads slowly to great abundance, and continued violation of her laws ends in desolation.

—Author Unknown

SPRINGTIDE FARE

THE BEST SPRING FOODS

By simply coordinating our diets with the cycles of the seasons, we naturally cleanse and build health for the body regardless of whether we choose to fast to cleanse and build, or eat to cleanse and build. By observing and practicing the basic principles that Nature teaches us, we come to understand that all of Nature is our classroom.

The plant kingdom provides not only body-building foods, calories, minerals, and vitamins essential for metabolic regulation,[6] but also "cleansing" foods that yield active substances employed as medicines. After a long winter of consuming the "building" foods needed for metabolism in the colder months, the body needs the fresh plant foods emerging in the spring to assist in the natural cleansing process to lighten itself for the warm days of summer.

The fundamental message of spring suggests renewal, repair, and cleansing by the very plant foods Nature sends forth at this time. Therefore, the primary foods to be enjoyed in spring and through summer should be mainly those for cleansing—the fresh vegetables, fruits, and herbs of the plant kingdom. Choose those that are locally grown and in season. If organic (grown without chemicals) foods cannot be found in your area, contamination can be minimized by soaking them (see food baths, chapter 5) and by juicing them. Most chemical contaminations are bound up in the fiber of plant foods; removing the fiber, in juicing, will render the foods more healthful. However, the "whole" vegetable and fruit are valuable in the diet, not only for their vitamins and minerals but also for the fiber, which tones and cleanses the inner intestinal system. Balance your diet with fiber foods and juices. In early spring we still draw upon winter root vegetables and squashes until the first fresh green vegetables appear. Among the latter are snow peas, artichokes, asparagus, and bitter lettuces. Fava beans, beets, and tender herbs follow. On the following pages you will find some of my favorite recipes for springtime eating, designed to facilitate your cleansing process.

BENEFICIAL SPRING FOODS

ORGANS: Liver, gallbladder
TIME: Spring
COLOR: Spring green
FRUITS: Kiwi, Valencia oranges, limes, grapefruit, and lemons (the most beneficial way to eat fruit is in its natural state). VEGETABLES: Asparagus, beets, sprouts, dandelion, chickweed, chicory, miner's lettuce, spring greens, parsley, broccoli, cabbage, cauliflower, daikon, wakame, sea palm, umeboshi, and sauerkraut. GRAINS: Barley, quinoa, wheat, millet, and rye.

FOODS THAT STRESS THESE ORGANS: Sugar and honey, fried foods, alcohol and drugs, coffee and chocolate, and excessive amounts of dairy and red meats.

❁ ENGLISH LAVENDER LEMONADE

The potent lemon is a valuable fruit for preserving health. As an antioxidant and cell membrane stabilizer, the vitamin C in lemons neutralizes harmful bacteria and is useful for liver restoration. In addition, this recipe is a fine example of how aromatic herbs will transform the flavor and nutritional value of an ordinary beverage. Its basic blend of dry herbs is reminiscent of the Victorian era when lavender was used for love and devotion, lemon balm for love and friendship, peppermint for virtue, and lemon verbena for sensibility. All of these herbs are known for their calming, antidepressant properties and healing effect on the lungs and liver. Spring, late summer, and autumn are all good seasons to enjoy the herbal and fruit lemonades offered here.

INGREDIENTS	AMOUNT
pure water	as directed
English lavender flowers	$1/4$ C.
lemon balm leaves	$3/4$ C.
peppermint leaves	$1/4$ C.
lemon verbena leaves	$3/4$ C.
lemon rind (organic or well scrubbed)	3 lemons
maple or brown rice syrup	$1/2$ C.
raw honey	$3/4$ C.
lemon juice (fresh)	$1^1/4$ C.

In a glass or stainless-steel pot, bring 8 cups water to boil; turn off heat. Add the dry herbs and cover tightly. Let stand for 8 hours or overnight; refrigerate when cool. Remove the zest of the 3 lemons with a paring knife, chop coarsely and combine with 2½ cups water in a saucepan. Cover and simmer (low heat) for 2 or 3 minutes. Remove from heat and allow to cool until lukewarm. Remove the zest and add the syrup and honey to the warm water, and stir until dissolved. Combine the sweet water and lemon juice to make a double-strength lemonade base. To serve, combine equal parts lemonade base, herbal tea, and water, adjusting taste as desired. Chill and serve in tall glasses or a punch bowl garnished with edible flowers, fresh herbs, or lemon slices. Lemonade base and herbal tea can be stored in covered glass jars for 3 or 4 days in the refrigerator. Serves 15 to 20.

✿ STRAWBERRY OR BLUEBERRY LEMONADE

Organically grown strawberries are a good source of iron, help to lower blood pressure and to detoxify the liver and kidneys. Berries and lemons are high in vitamin C and help to cleanse the stomach. Blue pigments, called anthocyanins, found in blue-berries, strawberries, and other blue-red fruits are potent antioxidants.

INGREDIENTS	AMOUNT
organic berries	½ C.
lemonade base (see above)	⅓ C.
pure water	2 C.
honey	1 T.

Combine berries and lemonade base. Blend until smooth, add water and honey. Chill lightly and serve with fruit garnish. Serves 1.

✿ DANDELION COOLER

Liquefy in a blender or juicer. Pour over ice, garnish with pineapple and fresh mint.

INGREDIENTS	AMOUNT
tender early-spring dandelion leaves	½ C.
unsweetened pineapple or apple juice	2 C.

✿ THE ENERGY BOMB BREAKFAST

The Energy Bomb is a potent blending of valuable enzymes and interrelated nutrients that are speedily assimilated by the glands to promote hormone vitality. It helps to stir up sleepy glands and boost the body-mind functions for the day.

Add whey powder to nutritional drinks to boost vitamin and mineral content. Whey powder is inexpensive and can be found at your natural foods store. Start with 1 tablespoon of powdered whey and work up to 3 times a day.

INGREDIENTS	AMOUNT
soy milk or oat milk (organic)	1 C.
raw almonds	3 to 6
vanilla extract	1 tsp.
nutmeg	$1/8$ tsp.
whey powder	1 T.
banana or apple (optional)	$1/4$

Combine all ingredients and blend vigorously. Serves 1.

CITRUS KISS

The Edgar Cayce health system recommends that we combine citrus fruits—orange, grapefruit, lemon, and lime—to strengthen the optical systems.[7] Clear, strong eyesight is a blessing worth its weight in gold. For many years, I have enjoyed these simple recipes and have maintained 20/20 vision. To receive the optimal benefit, citrus juices should be taken between meals or 1 to 2 hours before breakfast. However, they can be combined with an egg or whole wheat toast, but not cereal. Pink or ruby-red grapefruit offers up to 26 times more carotene content than the white variety.

❀ ORANGE OR GRAPEFRUIT KISS

Combine the ingredients and enjoy as directed above. Serves 1.

INGREDIENTS	AMOUNT
fresh-squeezed orange or grapefruit juice	$3/4$ C.
fresh-squeezed lemon or lime juice	$1/4$ C.

❀ PINEAPPLE KISS

The egg should be soft-boiled with a very runny yolk. Separate the yolk from the white. Combine the ingredients and blend to a frothy consistency. This drink is a real treat. Serves 1.

INGREDIENTS	AMOUNT
fresh pineapple juice	$3/4$ C.
egg yolk	1

PREPARING SALAD GREENS

The best salads are made with a good base mix of lettuce varieties such as red romaine, red mustard, green oak, or sorrel, and other greens such as amaranth, dandelion, arugula, and nasturtium leaves. Place the greens in a large bowl or sink full of cool water, and remove any damaged leaves. Swish slightly to remove any dirt, then wait a few minutes while the dirt settles to the bottom. To remove excess water, use a salad spinner or shake the leaves gently in a colander; salad dressings do not stick to wet leaves, so take extra care to dry them. Transfer the greens to a clean dry tea towel; roll up the towel and store in the refrigerator until you are ready to make your salad. For longer storage of washed greens, place them loosely in a covered glass bowl or jar with a few single paper towel sheets to absorb extra moisture. To prepare the salad, tear the greens into bite-size pieces. The dressing can be made fresh in the bowl; then put the greens on top and toss them together.

❀ SPIKE AND SPIRULINA SALAD SHAKE

The Aztecs in Mexico and native tribes in Central Africa highly valued the blue-green microalgae, spirulina, as a food. Spirulina, a descendant of the original life-form on Earth, has been replenishing itself for more than

INGREDIENTS	AMOUNT
spirulina or kelp	*1 oz.*
Spike	*2 oz.*

3.5 billion years. It contains the most powerful combination of unusual nutrients of any single grain, herb, or food. Spirulina is 60 to 70 percent highly digestible protein, 10 times higher in beta carotene than carrots, and has remarkably high levels of vitamins A and B12, iron, calcium, trace minerals, and RNA and DNA enzymes. It also contains chlorophyll, lysine, vitamin E, amino acids, and zinc! The most pleasant way I have found to consistently keep spirulina in my diet is to use it as a seasoning, which I have done for years; I cannot make a green salad without it. Try it and you will see why.

Spike is a trade name for an all-purpose, all-natural seasoning containing sea salt, yeast, vegetable protein, and powders of onion, celery, orange peel, garlic, dill, kelp, curry, horseradish, white pepper, savory, mustard, red and green bell pepper, parsley, tarragon, rose hip, saffron, mushroom, spinach, tomato, paprika, cayenne, oregano, basil, marjoram, rosemary, thyme, and lemon peel. It can usually be purchased inexpensively in bulk at natural foods stores. Its tendency to stick together is remedied by the addition of the spirulina. Combine the two well and store in a shaker bottle. Sprinkle on green salads and vegetable dishes. Spirulina and seasoning containing spirulina are best kept cool or refrigerated.

🌺 CARRIE'S KUMARI CURRY DRESSING

This is the salad dressing recipe that my friends and relatives always want. It is high in nutritional impact and big on flavor. Substitutions for the oils can be made, and varying amounts of apple cider vinegar, wine, or lemon juice can replace the aloe vera juice. Omega-3 essential fatty acids in the diet, such as those found here, may lower cho-

INGREDIENTS	AMOUNT
virgin olive oil	$^1/_3$ C.
flaxseed or hempseed oil (canola, avocado, pumpkin, or English walnut oil can be substituted)	$^1/_3$ C.
garlic clove (peeled)	1 whole
curry powder	$1^1/_2$ tsp.
dried tarragon, mint, dill, oregano thyme, marjoram, sage, rosemary, powdered turmeric, and powdered cumin	$^1/_2$ tsp. each
chopped capers	1 T.

lesterol levels and blood pressure, ease eczema and psoriasis, relieve arthritis inflammation, aid brain development, reduce cancer risk factors, prevent migraine headaches, and boost the immune system. Dr. Bronner's mineral bouillon and Bragg liquid aminos can replace tamari if desired. These all-purpose vegetable protein seasonings are highly nutritious and should find a place as valued cooking condiments in many dishes.

Put ingredients in a wide-mouth glass bottle or jar with a lid, and shake to coat herbs and spices with oils. (If possible, allow the spice and oil mixture to stand refrigerated for at least 2 hours to infuse oils with herbs. If time is short, omit this step and complete the dressing with the following.)

Combine these ingredients and incorporate with the oil and herbs. This is very good on salads and steamed vegetables. It can be combined with plain yogurt for variation. Keep all salad dressings refrigerated. Makes about $1^1/_2$ cups.

INGREDIENTS	AMOUNT
aloe vera juice or gel (or lemon juice, wine, or apple cider vinegar)	$^1/_3$ C.
prepared stone-ground mustard	$^1/_4$ C.
tamari	3 T.
maple syrup or molasses (optional)	1 tsp.

❦ TENDER DANDELION SALAD

Gather tender young dandelion leaves in early spring and wash them gently.

INGREDIENTS	AMOUNT
dandelion leaves	*3 C.*
olive oil	*2 T.*
flaxseed or canola oil	*2 T.*
apple cider vinegar	*2 T.*
fennel or anise seed	*1 tsp.*
fresh peppermint	*2 tsp.*
red onion	*2 thin slices*
tamari	*2 tsp.*
sweet honey mustard or miso	*2½ tsp.*

Combine the dressing ingredients and use as a topping for dandelion greens or lettuce combinations. A thick slice of whole grain bread such as rye, wheat, millet, oat, or corn is the perfect complement to this backyard banquet.

As the dandelion leaves become larger (and the days longer), gather a basketful; wash and steam them like spinach leaves. The crowns—those round, green knobs in the center of the young leaves—which in a few weeks rise on long stems to support a disc of bright yellow florets, can be steamed for 10 minutes and served with butter and whole grain breads. In early spring, when our bodies seem to cry out for fresh greens, the tender young dandelion is a welcome and invaluable restorative.

The taproot of dandelion, dug and dried in the autumn, is ready to be used as a medicinal tea (p. 213). A green drink is made by adding a handful of dandelion leaves to juice such as pineapple, for example, and blending well. Garnish with pineapple slice and mint.

SPRING SPROUTS

Eating sprouted foods will infuse your diet with the vital energy of spring. Adding sprouted seeds, beans, grains, and nuts will enliven many wonderful salads, vegetable sautés, and even nut milks. Sprouts are highly nutritional and good protein foods, many being complete proteins. As most sprouts grow, their protein content increases; when they become green, chlorophyll and many vitamins are being added, while the protein ratio decreases.

Almost any seed or bean will sprout; some favorites are alfalfa, sunflower, radish, and onion. Alfalfa seeds can be used alone or mixed with other good sprouters such as lentil, mung, garbanzo, and adzuki beans. Gelatinous seeds like flax and chia will not sprout well in a jar. Grains, peas, and some nuts such as raw almonds will sprout. The almond carries phosphorus and iron in a combination more easily assimilated than any other nut.

The seeds of amaranth, known to some gardeners as pigweed, are rich in high-quality protein, and both the seeds and the greens are loaded with calcium. Amaranth is one of the edible weeds commonly discarded by home gardeners who are unaware of its value.

SPROUTING SEED

1. Begin with a clean 1-quart glass jar and a very small wire mesh or cheesecloth. Use the rings of canning jar lids, rubber bands, or string to fasten the mesh or cheesecloth over the mouth of the jar. This allows for quick rinsing, drainage, and air circulation. If you want to make a large quantity of sprouts, use a 1-gallon jar and double the amount of seeds.

2. Choose organically grown seeds, grains, or legumes. Three beans that sprout easily are adzuki, mung, and lentil. Rinse the seeds in lukewarm water and remove any that are split or damaged.

3. Place 2 tablespoons seeds or ½ cup grains or legumes in the jar with 3 times as much water. Soak small seeds for 5 hours and seeds with very hard coats for up to 36 hours. Cress, oat, and mustard seeds do not need presoaking. The small wire mesh is best for draining small seeds. Switch to a larger screen after the sprouts become larger, for best drainage.

4. Rinse and drain the seeds twice a day, morning and evening. For well-drained seeds and sprouts, lay the jar at an angle; a warm dark place such as the cupboard is a good sprouting spot. Consider saving the nutritious rinse water you drain off to use in drinks, soups, sauces, or to water your plants.

5. After 3 or 4 days, when the sprouts are about 1-inch long, put them in the sunshine to green. After a day in the sun, they are ready to eat! If sunshine is scarce, omit this step and enjoy your sprouts in salads, soups, juices, casseroles, or other dishes.

❧ CURRIED EGGS WITH SPROUTS

Eggs are a symbolic springtime food. This dish can be enjoyed for breakfast, lunch, or dinner. Fresh sprouts surpass meat in nutritional value and lettuce and tomatoes in vitamin C. Sprouts are one of the few foods that contain vitamin B_{12} in abundance, plus a high amount of vitamin A.

Beat the eggs, water, curry, and

INGREDIENTS	AMOUNT
whole eggs	2
egg yolks	2
pure water	¼ C.
curry powder	1 tsp.
green onion or chives (sliced)	¼ C.
bean sprouts	2 C.
Spike Shake (p. 41)	optional
chili oil	optional

onion together; set aside. Chop the sprouts, put them in a heated iron skillet, and sprinkle them with water. Stir the sprouts and sprinkle them with Spike Shake if desired. Add the egg mixture and cook until the eggs are set but still moist (do not overcook). Stir the eggs gently and serve with a green salad if desired. Offer the chili oil as a condiment. Serves 2.

❁ CONFETTI CABBAGE SLAW

The healing chlorophyll in cabbage is a good springtime cleanser, and it also enriches the blood. Cabbage is rich in sulfur, calcium, and iodine, and it supplies nitrogen. There are many ways to utilize this valued vegetable. The following recipe is one of my favorites.

    Finely shred the cabbage and carrot, dice the peppers and onion, then combine all the ingredients except the beets. Toss the salad with the following dressing. Use beets as garnish if desired. Serves 6.

INGREDIENTS	AMOUNT
red cabbage	2 C.
green cabbage	2 C.
carrot (medium)	1
green and red bell peppers (combined)	1 C.
green onion or shallots	1/2 C.
raisins or currants (organic)	3/4 C.
caraway seeds	2 tsp.
sunflower seeds (optional)	2 T.
raw shredded beets	garnish

❁ DRESSING

Blend the ingredients to a creamy consistency and toss with the salad until evenly coated. This colorful side dish is good with the Asparagus and Quinoa Risotto (p. 49). Makes about 2/3 cup.

INGREDIENTS	AMOUNT
sour cream or plain yogurt	1/4 C.
mayonnaise (canola)	1/4 C.
apple cider vinegar or lemon juice	1 T.
prepared mustard	2 tsp.
apple juice	1 T.
dill weed	2 tsp.
paprika	1 tsp.
tamari	1/2 tsp.

❧ MISO SOUP WITH SUNCHOKES AND SHALLOTS

Like yogurt, miso is a living, cultured food that has an alkalizing effect on the body. It is basically made from soybeans, barley, water, sea salt, and fermented rice that has been aged for 3 years. This valuable energy food helps in the digestion and assimilation of other foods, absorbs and eliminates radioactive products from the system, and helps where air pollution

INGREDIENTS	AMOUNT
wakame (sea vegetable) 1½ inch strips	³/₄ C.
pure water	6 C.
bonito fish flakes	¹/₃ C.
sunchokes (diced)	1 C.
shallots (minced)	¹/₃ C.
red barley or hatcho miso	¹/₃ C.

is prevalent. In Japan, a warm cup of miso soup is used as a substitute for the morning cup of coffee for its energizing qualities, protein, vitamin B12, and other essential nutrients. The active properties in miso are destroyed if heated above 104 degrees F; it should be added to cooked foods just before serving. Traditional miso can be stored for months without refrigeration and will keep for more than a year if kept cool. Miso is always close at hand in my kitchen. It can become a flavorful soup in 10 minutes. The secret to making good miso soup is dried fish flakes, which are available at Asian markets.

Sunchokes (Jerusalem artichokes) are a natural form of insulin and contain valuable minerals as well as vitamins A, C, and B complex. This potato-like root vegetable tastes like a water chestnut when raw. It is recommended in many healing systems as a nutritious addition to your diet.

Rinse and soak the wakame for 30 minutes; save the liquid as stock. Bring the water and stock to a boil and add the fish flakes; lower heat and simmer 10 minutes. Dice the sunchokes, mince the shallots, and cut the wakame. Strain the fish flakes from the stock, return the stock to the soup pot, and reboil. Turn off the heat and add the veggies to the stock; cover tightly and set aside. Mix the miso paste with ½ cup of the warm stock and add it to the soup. Miso soup is nice garnished with chives or green onions and served with garlic bread. Try miso soup with mustard greens in summer, and with kale in winter. Serves 4.

❧ PITA PIZZA LA MEDITERRANEE

Pita pizzas are easy, elegant fare and adapt well to a variety of seasonal produce. This dish is inspired by a favorite neighborhood restaurant that offers fresh toppings from ratatouille to simple tomatoes and basil on pita pizzas. Served with a green salad and a dollop of hummus, this meal is a special treat. Round flat pita pocket bread is offered at most groceries. Choose good-quality whole wheat pita and store them in the freezer. When needed, toast the pitas to cut down on baking time. Cheese has calcium; choose goat, feta, and real Swiss for ease of digestibility.

INGREDIENTS	AMOUNT
asparagus tips	*8 to 12*
broccoli florets	*4*
whole wheat pita (8" rounds)	*4*
olive oil	*2 T.*
red onion (sliced thin)	*4 slices*
feta and ricotta cheeses	*1/2 C. each*
Swiss cheese (sliced very thin)	*4 slices*
fresh garlic, oregano, and basil	*to season*
fresh parsley	*garnish*

Wash, cut, and steam the asparagus and broccoli until crunchy tender. Toast the pita, brush one side of each bread with olive oil, spread with ricotta, and sprinkle evenly with feta. Season with herbs and top with separated rings of onion and veggies. Top the veggies with one slice of Swiss cheese per pizza and sprinkle with parsley. Place the pizzas under the broiler for about 5 minutes or until the cheese melts. Serve whole or cut into quarters and arrange on plate with a green salad and hummus if desired. Serves 4.

QUINOA

If you have never tried quinoa, spring is the perfect time to enjoy this light, unique, and versatile food. Quinoa, pronounced "keen-wa," is called the Mother Grain by the people of the Andes. The Incas deemed the kernels sacred, since a steady diet appeared to ensure long lives.

The name quinoa was reputedly tagged on the innocent grain by Francisco Pizarro himself, shortly after he and his army straggled into the Incas' stronghold at Cuzco in 1532. According to Peruvian lore, once Pizarro tasted a bowl of cooked quinoa, he demanded to see where this seed grew. When he had climbed the Andean plateau and studied the plants' tall stalks and brilliant blossoms lightly dusted with snow, the conquistador is said to have murmured, "Quimera!" (Fantastic). He called it "the grain that grows where grass will not."

Pizarro realized that the highly sophisticated Indian culture represented a threat to Spanish colonization. He banned the growing of quinoa in the mountains and had the Incas plant formal vegetable gardens instead. The tender greens shriveled as the first blast of icy Andean wind hit the altiplano, but Pizarro refused to be discouraged. He imported

Spanish livestock to graze in the lower valleys so the Incas would learn to eat meat and reject their "God-given" comestibles like potatoes, corn, and quinoa.

But the Incas were strict vegetarians, so the cattle languished and the sheep lay down with the llamas. Not allowed to grow quinoa, the Incas ate wild mushrooms instead. After years of raiding the altiplano, where he suspected quinoa still grew "under cover," Pizarro developed weak lungs and a cough that turned his once booming voice into a faint whisper. Wherever he looked, he saw defeat, and eventually he took the remnants of his army and left Peru forever.

Technically quinoa is not a grain at all; agrobotanists dub it a dried fruit of the *Chenopodium* herb family—whose best-known member is a wild and spicy green known as lamb's quarters.[8] Like lamb's quarters, quinoa's leaves are edible and delicious in a salad bowl. This is a food to savor.

Quinoa is cultivated for its copious seeds. A cup of cooked quinoa is equal to a quart of milk in calcium content, and it is very high in protein. All quinoa is not equal; as a general rule, look for the largest, whitest grains you can find. Quinoa seeds are naturally coated with saponin (a built-in insect repellent), and are slightly sticky, somewhat acid to the tongue, and foamy when wet. Most saponin is scrubbed off quinoa before it is dried and packaged, but the flavor of cooked quinoa will depend largely on how much rinsing you do. The more you rinse, the milder the flavor. Fully cooked quinoa is completely transparent and has a small white sprout, or tail, that surrounds the seed.

Quinoa's natural oiliness makes it a prime target for spoilage; even under the best conditions—below 65 degrees F—its shelf life is never longer than a month, and less if the mercury rises. Quinoa is extremely easy to prepare; it requires only about 12 to 15 minutes to cook. Do not pressure-cook it, since it may clog the pressure release valve.

❁ BASIC QUINOA

In a medium saucepan, heat the water or stock. Rinse the quinoa under cold water several times; drain. Combine the quinoa with the heated liquid and bring to a boil. Reduce heat to medium-low,

INGREDIENTS	AMOUNT
vegetable or chicken stock or water	*1 C.*
quinoa	*½ C.*
butter (organic)	*1 T.*

cover, and cook until the liquid is absorbed and the quinoa looks transparent, 12 to 15 minutes. Toss in butter (optional) and blend with a fork. Serves 2.

Note: Toasting quinoa in a dry skillet, after rinsing but prior to cooking, will bring out the full-bodied flavor. Sauté it with a small minced onion, finely chopped carrot, or a handful of cut herbs, to change its flavor and texture. Rosemary is a wonderful herb to add to quinoa.

❧ SPRING ASPARAGUS AND QUINOA RISOTTO

Quinoa is considered the number one whole protein cereal by the United Nations World Health Organization. This recipe is enhanced by the most tender spring asparagus tips, high in vitamin A and a good blood builder. I like to serve this atop a bed of fresh greens with a bit of Kumari Curry Dressing (p. 42).

INGREDIENTS	AMOUNT
quinoa	1½ C.
onion (finely chopped)	1½ C.
vegetable or chicken broth	3 C.
asparagus tips	15 to 20
butter (organic)	2 T.
curry paste or powder	1 T.
tamari	1 T.
fresh chives (finely chopped)	⅓ C.
apples and currants (chopped)	garnish

Rinse the quinoa well as directed in the basic recipe. Over low heat, simmer the onion in 2 tablespoons broth for about 5 minutes. Add the quinoa, mix well, and gently simmer for another 2 minutes. Add remaining broth and simmer in a covered pot until the quinoa is tender, about 20 minutes. Cut the asparagus tips in half, if they are large; add them to the pot with the quinoa and stir gently. Cover tightly and remove from heat. In a separate saucepan, gently melt the butter, add the curry paste or powder, and stir until incorporated. Blend the spice mixture with the quinoa and add the tamari and fresh chives. Serve this on a bed of greens with a garnish of apples or currants for a bit of sweetness, if desired. Serves 4 to 6.

❧ PASTA GARAM MASALA

Garam masala ("heating spices") is a spice blend that forms the basis of many Unani Tibb dishes. Unani Tibb refers to the system of medicine that was developed in the late tenth and early eleventh century by the famous physician Hakim Ibn Sina, called Avicenna in the West. There are quite a few different blends of garam masala available. To make your own, mix equal parts powdered ginger, cumin, coriander, and cinnamon with ½ part powdered nutmeg and red pepper. To make curry powder, make up garam masala and add 1 part turmeric and ½ part fenugreek and black mustard seeds. Pesto recipes can be found on pages 82 and 167.

In a large skillet, sauté the onion in the wine or broth for 5 minutes and add the diced vegetables. Sauté for 10 minutes. While the veggies are cooking, add the pasta to boiling water, breaking it in half and sprinkling it over the boiling bubbles. Cook the pasta until just tender (not soggy) and drain. To the veggies, add the garam masala, minced basil, and cilantro. Stir and sauté for 2 more minutes.

INGREDIENTS	AMOUNT
yellow onion (diced)	1¼ C.
white wine or broth	⅓ C.
zucchini or seasonal mixed veggies	4 C.
whole grain spelt pasta (organic)	¾ lb.
garam masala	2¼ tsp.
fresh basil and cilantro (minced)	2 T. each
basil or rosemary pesto	¾ C.
smoked salmon, tofu, or tempeh (optional)	½ C.
freshly shredded Parmesan (organic)	garnish

Adjust the heat to low and stir in the pesto. Add the cooked pasta and toss until well combined. Add the optional ingredients if desired. Garnish with shredded Parmesan and serve with a large green salad. Fantastic! Serves 4 to 6.

❀ PINEAPPLE MANDARIN TAPIOCA

Pineapples contain pepsin, which aids digestion and helps to regulate the glands. Pineapple and mandarin oranges contain high doses of blood-purifying vitamins C and B complex, and minerals. Tapioca is from the manioc root, grown in the tropics, and nutritious for its folic acid and manganese content.

INGREDIENTS	AMOUNT
pearl tapioca	½ C.
pure water	½ C.
pineapple juice	1 C.
orange juice	½ C.
maple or brown rice syrup	⅓ C.
pineapple chunks	1½ C.
mandarin orange sections	1 C.
heavy cream or plain yogurt	½ C.
vanilla extract	1 tsp.

Soak the tapioca in the water for 10 minutes and bring to a simmer for 10 minutes. Remove from heat and stir in the fruit juices and syrup. Dice the fruit and whip the cream. When the tapioca mixture has cooled, stir in the vanilla and fold in the cream or yogurt and fruit. Serves 4.

❀ EASY VANILLA MILLET PUDDING

Millet is always on hand in my kitchen. Once you start to use this versatile grain, you may have a cup or two left over from time to time. Millet is so valuable in the diet that it should be prepared for breakfast or lunch, dinner, or even dessert! You will find other good recipes for keeping millet in the diet in these chapters. Here is one that works well for breakfast, a snack, or dessert.

INGREDIENTS	AMOUNT
raisins or currants	1 T.
dried figs (diced)	2 T.
millet (toasted and cooked)	1½ C.
cinnamon or vanilla bean seeds	1 tsp.
water	1¼ C.
maple or rice syrup (optional)	1 T.
kuzu root starch	1 T.
cold water	2 T.
flaxseed or pine nuts (ground)	2 tsp.
vanilla extract	1 tsp.
dried apricots (diced)	2 T.
yellow delicious apples (diced)	1½ C.

In a saucepan, simmer the raisins, figs, and millet with the cinnamon, 1¼ cups water, and syrup for 10 to 15 minutes. Dissolve the kuzu in 2 tablespoons cold water and stir in until the pudding thickens. Grind the flaxseed to a meal and stir it in with all remaining ingredients. Serve warm. Serves 2.

CHAPTER FOUR

SUMMER RESTORATION

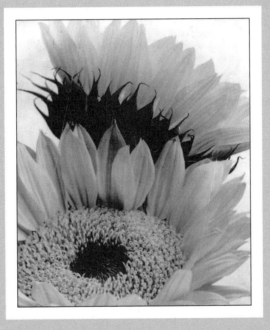

WE RECEIVE OUR ENERGY BY EATING THE
SUNLIGHT IN PLANTS AND ANIMALS. EVERY
HEARTBEAT AND EVERY STEP YOU TOOK
TODAY WAS FUELED BY THE SUN.[1]

—ELIOT COWAN

SUMMER

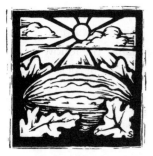

It is no small wonder that Nature provides us with such an abundance of water-filled fruits and vegetables when our bodies are most in need of them. The heavy heat of summer gives us an intuitive urge to eat lightly, keep it light, and become light.

Summer is associated with the Fire element. The **heart** and **small intestine** are ruled by this element, as are the functions of circulation and heating in the body.

Diet and exercise are very important to keep the Fire element strong, just as proper nutrition is vital to maintain a healthy heart while providing fuel and heat for the body. With such an abundance of fresh foods in summer, it is easier to cut back on—or eliminate—more of the refined foods and animal fats, particularly red meats, dairy products, and other fatty foods. This allows the small intestine to cleanse itself and lightens the load on the heart.

THE SMALL INTESTINE

The proper functioning of the small intestine is key to our nourishment because we digest and assimilate nutrients through its 23-foot-long carpet of villi.[2] The small intestine connects the stomach to the large intestine. It is divided into three parts: the duodenum, the jejunum, and the ileum.

As the digested food particles are spread upon the intestinal carpet of villi for absorption, the quantity and the quality of the food material are very important. Rich, fatty, difficult-to-digest foods make up 40 percent of the average North American diet. Villi have no regulating mechanism to indicate how much to absorb, so the result is that we can become either obese or ill. Other problems arise from foods we eat that act as glue to the delicate villi. Among these "glues" are chocolate (unfortunately!), hydrogenated peanut butter, processed cheeses, fried foods, and white flour products, to name a few. But this is not news in modern society.

When the body chemistry is abnormal because of the ingestion of food that ferments or putrefies in the small intestine, the resulting products are irritating to the delicate lining of the bowel. The bowel either tries to alleviate the irritation quickly—which results in diarrhea—or puts a spastic clamp on the intestines to keep the peristalsis from proceeding further—resulting in stasis or constipation.

✿ CLEANSE AND TONE THE SMALL INTESTINE

There are ways to clean the intestinal tract with herbal brooms (see below) or scrubbers such as marsh mallow and pepsin, black walnut, psyllium hulls and seeds, bran, slippery elm, bentonite, flaxseed, chia seed, and alfalfa. The following cleansing diet for the small intestine will acquaint you with some of these super foods. You will be surprised at how good they taste. I like to cleanse the digestive system before starting any fast. Use the Epsom Salts or Castor Oil internal baths in chapter 7 for best results.

TIME: Summer
TIME FRAME: 2 weeks

DAYS 1 AND 2: In the morning, do a skin brush and cleanse the digestive tract (chapter 7). By 3 or 4 P.M., after the digestive system has been sufficiently emptied, begin to take the Papaya Smoothies (p. 56). Papaya is especially full of digestive enzymes. The Center for Science in the Public Interest ranked papaya number one over 39 other fruits for its vitamins A and C, potassium, fiber, and carotenoid content. The drink works to soften excess mucus and blockage in the small intestine.

✿ INTESTINAL BROOM POWDER

This broom powder is used in the Papaya Smoothie recipe on page 56. Grind these ingredients to a powder in a blender or nut grinder. Have a total of 5 drinks per day, spaced 3 hours apart, and drink water and herbal teas in between.

INGREDIENTS	AMOUNT
psyllium seed	2 T.
chia seed	2 T.
flaxseed	2 T.
fenugreek seed	1 tsp.
slippery elm powder	2 T.
oat bran	2 T.
marsh mallow root	1 T.

✿ PAPAYA SMOOTHIE

Put the papaya, apple juice, water, nutmeg, and broom powder in the blender and puree. Take one pepsin tablet with each smoothie and drink water, clear vegetable broth, or herbal teas in between them. For dinner eat dried figs.

INGREDIENTS (per drink)	AMOUNT
fresh papaya	$1/3$ C.
fresh apple juice	$1/2$ C.
pure water	$1/2$ C.
nutmeg	$1/8$ tsp.
Intestinal Broom Powder (p. 55)	$1 1/2$ tsp.
pepsin tablet	1

DAYS 3 THROUGH 7: For breakfast, choose from the Breakfast Seed Cereal (below), seasonal fruit, or Papaya Smoothie. Drink the smoothies three hours apart, with fresh-pressed vegetable juices or clear vegetable broth in between. For lunch and dinner, along with the figs have $1/2$ to 1 cup brown rice and lentils (p. 57). This diet will begin to sweep clean the whole digestive tract, after the Papaya Smoothies have done the softening work.

✿ BREAKFAST SEED CEREAL

This cereal is a tasty, concentrated dish offering a treasure trove of hormone-stimulating nutrients and roughage to tone the whole intestinal system. Have this food for breakfast or lunch as specified.

Grind seeds and nuts to a fine meal in a blender or nut grinder. Place this mixture in a bowl; add raisins and enough apple juice to

INGREDIENTS	AMOUNT
flaxseed	1 tsp.
sesame seed	1 T.
sunflower seed	1 T.
raw almonds	1 T.
chia seed	1 T.
raisins or currants (organic)	1 to 2 T.
fresh raw apple juice	to cover

cover the seed mixture. Cover and allow to stand overnight (do not refrigerate); it will be ready to eat in the morning. As a rule in recipes, choose organic raisins or currants because grapes, as a crop, are generally treated with pesticides. Serves 2.

DAYS 8 THROUGH 14: Gradually return to a normal healthy diet. Add vegetable salads and whole grain foods. For the next 7 to 10 days, continue to have the Papaya Smoothies for breakfast, and include the brown rice and lentils for lunch or dinner along with a green salad. A small amount of tamari and Spike Shake may be used to flavor the brown rice and lentils.

✿ BROWN RICE AND LENTILS

This food combination, to cleanse and tone the small intestine, comes from herbalist William LeSassier. It will also improve body heat, diges-tion, and assimilation. Enjoy this food for lunch or dinner as specified.

INGREDIENTS	AMOUNT
brown rice	1/2 C.
lentils	1/2 C.
sunflower seeds	1/2 C.
pure water	2 1/2 C.

Simmer ingredients slowly for about 45 minutes or until tender. Eat 1 or 2 cups daily for a few weeks. It is a tasty, filling dish, and a great metabolic heat producer.

✿ SUMMER BLOOD CLEANSER

Help your heart to function optimally during the summer months by cleansing your blood. This will benefit all the tissues in the body. Eat this diet for a mini-mum of 3 days or a maximum of 10 days. This cleansing diet is based on European folk medicine, and it works like a charm.

TIME: Summer
TIME FRAME: 3 to 10 days

Put 2 heaping tablespoons of flaxseed in 6 cups pure water, boil for 30 min-utes, and strain. Drink the flaxseed tea warm or cool, mixed with a combination of fresh-pressed beet, carrot, and apple juice in the proportion of 2 parts tea to 1 part juice. Enjoy the tea throughout each day until you have consumed 32 ounces, or 1 quart.

1. For breakfast: fresh seasonal fruit.
2. For lunch: salad and vegetables with cold-pressed oil dressing and herbs.
3. For dinner: plain yogurt combined with vegetable puree and herbs, butter-milk, rice, vegetables, and echinacea tea.

✿ SENECA INDIAN SUMMER CLEANSING DIET

For North American Indian tribes, the practice of fasting and utilizing seasonal cleansing diets was a natural way to harmonize the body, mind, and spirit with all of Nature. The following comes from the Seneca Indians and is adapted from the books *Good Health Through Special Diets* by Hanna Kroeger and *Health Handbook* by Louise Tenney.

TIME: Summer
TIME FRAME: 4 days

DAY 1: All the fruit you want: apples, berries, watermelon, peaches, cherries, apricots, and so forth. No bananas, however.

DAY 2: All the herbal tea you want: gentian, Irish moss, cascara sagrada, goldenseal, comfrey, fenugreek, safflower, myrrh, yellow dock, echinacea, black walnut, barberry, dandelion, buchu, chickweed, catnip, and cyani—combined to help cleanse the whole system. Or choose your favorites, peppermint perhaps, or chamomile. Prepare a Standard Medicinal Tea as on page 213.

DAY 3: All the vegetables you want: steamed, raw, roasted, and baked.

DAY 4: Prepare a big pot of vegetable broth. Use pure water and boil all your leftover vegetables, adding others if needed to create a delicious mineral-rich soup. Potatoes, peas, corn, onion, carrots, broccoli, green pepper, zucchini, cabbage, and parsley are good possibilities along with green beans and summer squash. Season the broth with Bragg Aminos or Dr. Bronner's Mineral Bouillon. Drink the broth only; strain out the vegetables, which may be eaten after the fourth day.

   This diet cleanses the colon on the first day. It releases toxins, salt, and excessive calcium deposits in the muscles, tissues, and organs on day two. The digestive tract is supplied with mineral-rich bulk on day three. The blood, lymph, and inner organs are mineralized on day four.

SIMPLE JUICE FASTING

In various detoxifying regimes, juices have played an important part. The purposes of a diet restricted to juices are:

1. To flush the system with large amounts of liquid.
2. To "rest" the digestive organs. Because juices of vegetables and fruits contain very little protein, the body is relieved of the multitudinous and complex processes of digesting the food. The sugars are in most cases of the most simple structure and need no

digestion at all. And the fact that there is little or no fat or oil in the majority of fruits and vegetables eliminates the necessity of this type of digestion for a time.

3. To supply food that is low in acid ash. Proteins and fats are the two types of foods that, when used by the body, result in an acid ash.

4. To reduce the putrefactive processes. Proteins are the only food elements that putrefy, so it is easy to see that, on a juice diet, putrefaction is lessened. This lessening of the putrefactive processes also reduces the production of purine and uric acid.

5. To reduce the fermentative activity. Starches and sugars are the only two food elements that ferment. Complex sugars and large amounts of starch often ferment, resulting in gas formation in the stomach and also in the 23 feet of small intestine. Juices supply very little starch, and their sugars are usually of a simple structure. Requiring no digestion, these do not linger in the stomach to ferment but are readily absorbed into the blood.

6. To supply those elements necessary to maintain the alkalinity of the tissues. Juices, especially if the entire vegetable or fruit is used, abound in those minerals—sodium, potassium, calcium, magnesium—whose function is to maintain an alkaline balance. However, it must be remembered that the richest source of these minerals is immediately beneath the fruit or vegetable skin. So, if the potatoes or beets or apples are peeled, much valuable mineral supply is wasted. In using a good juicer, all of the fruit or vegetable is used, and no minerals are wasted. A good kitchen juicer is a valuable tool for keeping fresh juices in the daily diet. A manual juicer that crushes the cells of the fibers of vegetables and fruits is recommended, or a triturator type such as the Champion, Vita Mix, or the German-engineered AEG Juicer (see Sources). The expense involved is an investment in your health that pays for itself.

SPECIAL TIMES FOR JUICE FASTING

Spring and summer are the best times for major cleansing and for fasting on liquids for a period of 1 to 10 days or longer. You may develop a schedule of fasting for only 1 day per week or a 3-day period monthly. This fasting will indeed strengthen, lengthen, and lighten your life—preventing physical degeneration by eliminating toxic buildup in tissues and organs, allowing rest to the systems, and facilitating proper physiology.

Those who wish to do a long liquid cleanse (30 days or more), or who have acute or chronic illnesses, should have professional supervision—though it is rare to have any difficulty other than lack of willpower in a juice cleanse or fast of any kind.

A 1-day fast can be very healing and should not be underestimated as a health rejuvenator. It should last for a period of 24 hours. The best days to fast in any week are Thursday, Friday, and Monday, which are the "Days of Excellence" according to the Sufis. The best days to fast in any month are the first, middle, and last days of every month. In addition, there can be fasting on the thirteenth, fourteenth, and fifteenth days of the moon's cycle.

Fasting 2 days or more could begin on any of the above-mentioned days. Friday is particularly good, especially if you are working a 9-to-5 weekly job schedule. The week-end serves as a mini-fasting vacation that can easily be extended to Monday and beyond, since by this time you will know your comfort level with it and be in control.

If you seek to renew and transform the blood through a cleansing fast, the 10-day fasting period is most effective. Human blood decomposes and is renewed every day at the rate of 300 million globules per second—or one-tenth of the total blood supply each day. Therefore, the blood should be entirely transformed and renewed in 10 days.

If you suffer with allergies or frequent colds, these cleanses will help relieve symptoms and clear toxins and excess mucus from your body. Any of the internal and external baths (chapter 7) are excellent additions to juice fasting.

JUICE FASTING ESSENTIALS

If the whole fruit or vegetable, including the peel, seeds, and core, is liquefied through a juicer, if it is made fresh each time, and if this liquid is balanced with the juices of deep green leaves, it will provide all the food elements needed to carry on normal metabolism. If a long juice fast is undertaken, I like to take a teaspoon or two of fresh flaxseed oil or hempseed oil daily with the juice. The essential amino acids in these oils are cleansing and keep the immune system strong.

Pectin is Nature's fruit laxative, and too much of this is lost when the peel is not eaten. Many people who find an apple to be laxative in action fail to obtain that effect from apple juice or cider as commonly used. The grape is another fruit supplying much pectin. Pectin and cellulose can be obtained in whole fresh juices, along with all of the protective elements, vitamins, and minerals. For these reasons, juices are important supplements as daily additions to any diet.

The reasons for juice diets are many. Foods that may be underlying causes of disease are eliminated. Foods that are difficult or slow to digest are eliminated. Foods that are constipating are eliminated. Foods that throw a burden on the liver and gallbladder are eliminated. Foods that demand too much from the pancreas are eliminated. Foods that leave toxic waste are eliminated. Foods that cause gas formation are eliminated. Foods that carry disease-forming bacteria and parasites into the body are eliminated. Foods that are acid-forming are eliminated. So, in truth, this diet has come to be known as the Eliminating Diet.

Juice fasting is highly cleansing and detoxifying because wastes that have been held in the stomach and colon for a long time may at last empty. Many digestive troubles have been overcome by this simple process of emptying the stomach. Many people never empty their stomachs; they eat too much to dispose of it between feedings, ingesting too many slow-to-digest foods and selecting too many unhealthful hard-to-digest foods. Such holdovers ferment and produce stomach gas, with its attendant belching and other distressing symptoms that continue throughout the intestinal tract.

Raw, fresh juices contain wonderful chemicals called "enzymes" that are a great aid in the digestion of other foods. Then there are other enzymes made by the body, and these juices stimulate that enzyme flow. Enzymes also aid in preparing other food substances, such as protein, for use by the body. Many enzymes normally present in raw fruit and vegetables are destroyed by cooking, which is one more reason for the inclusion of raw juices in a cleansing regimen and in the daily diet.

WHEY POWDER

Whey powder is an excellent addition to fresh juices to aid in the assimilation of nutrients. Whey is a mild residue left over from cheese making. It helps to feed the beneficial bacteria in the intestines and prevents the development of harmful putrefactive bacteria. Whey helps to prevent constipation, internal sluggishness, and gas and bowel putrefaction when used regularly. It contains rich amounts of B complex vitamins, especially B_1 and B_2, which are very important for preserving a youthful appearance and preventing premature aging. Start with 1 tablespoon a day and work up to 3 times a day.

JUICES FOR REDUCING WEIGHT

Most fresh fruit and vegetable juices are low in calories. So, a simple exchange of high-calorie foods (such as starches, sugars, and fats) for low-calorie juices will provide a good basis for a weight-reducing plan. It is most advisable to include the juices in every reducing diet because these diets may seriously diminish the supply of protective elements. By using fresh-pressed juices several times a day, you may be sure of obtaining those two must-haves—vitamins and minerals.

SUMMER SOLSTICE SOJOURN

If you are fasting for the first time, it is a good idea to choose a simple regimen like the following recipe. The ingredients needed for the Fasting Juice are easily obtained and available throughout the summer months in most areas. Make sure the vegetables, fruits, and herbs have been organically grown without exposure to any pesticides or chemicals. This recipe will yield about 2 quarts and will last two people two days. However, the nutrient content of the juice is best when it is made fresh each day and consumed within one or two hours after pressing.

✿ SUMMER SOLSTICE FASTING JUICE

Take the pits out of the avocados and scoop out the flesh into a blender jar. Put the remaining vegetables through a juicer, then add them to the avocados, and blend. Take 1 tablespoon cold-pressed olive oil twice daily while on the juice; blend the oil into the juice. Makes about 2 quarts.

INGREDIENTS	AMOUNT
ripe avocados	2
fresh red tomatoes (large)	2
carrots (with tops)	2 bunches
celery	12 stalks
yellow summer squash	3
burdock root	1 tsp.
red beets (small)	2
pure water	2 C.

1. For the first 5 days, drink only the juice and eat no other foods. Space each 8- to 10-ounce drink 2 or 3 hours apart and drink pure distilled water and lemon juice in between. Before bedtime drink chamomile or peppermint tea.

   The use of enemas and colonics is very beneficial during this fast. Be sure to use filtered water so that you do not introduce any water-borne parasites—such as *Giardia*—into your digestive system. Acidophilus capsules should be taken in conjunction with colonics to restore the natural "good" bacteria of the intestines. Acidophilus can also be introduced into the lower bowel by breaking open a capsule and including the powder in the enema water. A normal healthy digestive system does not require enemas on a daily basis. Overuse of enemas can impair the natural function of the bowels.

2. At the end of 5 days on the vegetable juice, go on a pure water and lemon juice fast for another 5 days. One teaspoon of fresh lemon juice is added to 8- to 10-ounces of pure water.

3. After 5 days of lemon and water fasting, follow with 3 more days on the fasting vegetable juice, then add simple salads and whole grains for another 3 days.

This fast is a lifesaver when the body is exhausted from too much traveling, too many restaurant meals, or too many late work nights. The atmosphere in which you do a fast is important: no stress, no strenuous workouts, meditate daily, and take time for renewal and relaxation.

✿ SUMMER FRUIT PUNCH

This juice combination has a rich supply of vitamins and minerals that boosts the health of the glands; it can be enriched by the addition of gelatin if desired. This juice works quickly to rid the body of excess fat and mucus.

INGREDIENTS	AMOUNT
berry juice	¼ C.
grape juice	¼ C.
apple juice	¼ C.
lemon juice	2 T.
whey powder	1 T.
unflavored gelatin (optional)	1 or 2 T.

Combine the fruit juices in equal proportions, add lemon juice and whey. Dissolve gelatin in 1 cup hot water and add to each quart of juice if desired. Drink this juice combination for a minimum of 1 day—anytime you are hungry. Eat no solid food or other foods but take a multivitamin every day if desired. Be sure to keep the intestinal tract clear with a laxative herbal remedy each day, or do enema therapy.

JUICES FOR GAINING WEIGHT

When a person is chronically thin and noticeably underweight, two things are usually required to reverse the condition: First, the reason for inadequate assimilation of foods must be found and corrected. Then, weight-gaining foods must be added. The most common cause of underweight in the apparently healthy individual lies in the intestines, where two primary conditions may be preventing normal assimilation. These are constipation and intestinal mucus. These conditions are eradicated by employing a colon-cleansing fast, along with special herbs and juices to cleanse the small intestine and digestive tract; then high-calorie juices are added to build up the body. The juices include wonderful blends of liquefied fruits, nuts, and vegetable oils: banana-nut shakes (wherein the whole banana is converted into a liquid), fancy-flavored organic soybean milks (with their fine supply of soybean oil), and luscious sweet drinks of natural sugar, rich organic raisins, dates, and figs. These are but a few of the healthful drinks for the weight seeker.

✿ WEIGHT SEEKER COLADA

Slice the frozen banana and place it in
a blender with the remaining ingredients. Process until creamy, and enjoy
as an addition to a balanced diet.
Adjust the amounts to taste. Serves 1.

INGREDIENTS	AMOUNT
frozen banana (whole)	1
fresh cream	2 T.
coconut milk or apple juice	¼ C.
fresh pineapple	⅓ C.
almonds (raw)	3 to 6
sugarless raspberry jam (optional)	1 T.

JUICES FOR THE CONVALESCING OR AGED

Juices are especially adapted for the diets of convalescents and the aged. They are both satisfying and comforting to the old and sick who often lack the energy, if not the teeth, to
chew sufficient solid foods. Juices can be served warm to impart a nourishing internal
glow. A variety of fresh-pressed juices will supply all the needed factors.

PREGNANCY AND NURSING

Scarcity of mother's milk can in most instances be traced to poor dietary habits in the
months just prior to delivery. Raw, fresh juices, in variety, contain all the elements necessary for ample milk production.

SELECTING YOUR JUICES

To obtain all of the elements and values discussed, the juices must be made of live, raw
foods—not canned, bottled, pasteurized, or preserved. Canned and bottled juices contain
few or none of the protective elements needed by the body to maintain health. Every
household should be equipped for making fresh juices that are taste sensations. Cocktails
and broths can be made by liquefying basic foods such as vegetables, fruits, nuts, grains,
leaves, seeds, beans, peas, herbs, and oils. Create your own delicious combinations to suit
your taste. The benefits of juicing are worth the expense. For people who cannot afford a
juicer, organic foods should be eaten.

CARROT JUICE

The carrot, first cousin to ginseng, is an excellent base for delightful juice combinations
for fasting. Carrots are rich in beta-carotene and have proven anticancer activity. Foods

with carotenoids are highly effective as antioxidants and immune stimulators. The carotene is easily absorbed by the body when vegetables are liquefied or juiced, but the juice should be consumed immediately after juicing as much of this vitamin is destroyed by oxygen. Include the portion close to the top of carrots; it may appear harder and less desirable, but it carries the vital energies that stimulate the optical reactions between the kidneys and the eyes.

Note: The pulp from juiced carrots is exceptionally useful in treating mumps and tonsillitis if applied externally; use as a plaster to the throat and leave it on until dry.

These are delicious carrot juice combinations made in a ratio of $1^1/_4$ cups carrot juice to $^1/_2$ cup other juices:

- carrot - fresh horseradish
- carrot - apple - parsley
- carrot - celery - parsley
- carrot - celery - beet
- carrot - cucumber - parsley
- carrot - apple - ginger ($^1/_4$ inch piece)
- carrot - yam - ginger ($^1/_4$ inch piece)

Note: 1 to 2 tablespoons of whey powder can be added to carrot juices.

✸ "ENERGY FLUSH" JUICE FAST

Clark Gable used this recipe during the filming of *Gone with the Wind.* This juice is good when fasting for 1 to 4 days. It flushes out fat, gives instant energy, and rids the body of poisons. It may be incorporated with other fasts that allow extra juices.

Mix this juice combination with an equal part of pure water. Drink within 1 hour. An herbal laxative tea (chapter 7) should accompany this juice fast. Since fresh-pressed juices should not stand too long before being consumed, use this as a rejuvenating "day off" or "weekend" fast.

INGREDIENTS	AMOUNT
carrots	2
green beans	$^1/_2$ C.
parsley	$^1/_2$ C.
celery	$1^1/_2$ stalks
spinach	$^1/_2$ C.
gingerroot or horseradish	$^1/_2$ inch
apple	1

✿ GELATIN JUICE FAST
TIME: SUMMER
TIME FRAME: 1 to 10 days

INGREDIENTS	AMOUNT
gelatin granules	*1 T.*
hot water	*⅓ C.*
fresh raw vegetable juice	*8 to 10 oz.*
kelp powder or liquid	*¼ tsp.*

Gelatin is a highly beneficial gland food because it is a prime source of nearly all the essential amino acids or metabolized protein needed to feed your endocrine glands. The glands take up the amino acids from the gelatin and use them to nourish the blood, enrich the tissues, rejuvenate the organs, smooth the skin, nourish the hair, and feed the fibers of the nails. Their hormones feed the nerves and brain and help promote a healthful feeling of overall improvement in body and mind. The hormones themselves are composed of the very same amino acids found in gelatin. The protein hormones work to create gamma globulin, a blood protein that forms antibodies, which neutralize bacteria, viruses, and other microorganisms.

Dissolve the gelatin in the hot water, combine with juice and add kelp; drink 4 servings per day. If you are fasting on juices only, spread the gelatin juice cocktails out—one in the morning, at noon, and in the evening—and drink juices without gelatin in between. Gelatin juice cocktails are very good to add to the daily diet for extra nourishment and to strengthen the immune system.

Note: Gelatin is made from animal-derived products.

THE HEART

In Chinese folk medicine, it is said that the condition of the heart may be read from the color of a person's complexion, body, and especially the fingertips and the skin under the fingernails (red, pink, blue, white). The tongue should be moist and pink. If it is red, then the Fire or heart energy may be too strong, making it hard to relax or slow down. If the tongue is pale, it may reflect weakness of the Fire element, or possible anemia—a reduction of circulating red blood cells that lessens the capacity of the blood to carry oxygen and nutrients throughout the body. There are many causes of anemia, but all affect the amount of circulating oxygen, and thus can create symptoms like lethargy, slowness in action and thought, and coldness, especially in the hands and feet. A coated tongue relates more to diet and poor digestive functioning. If a person smokes, a yellow-coated tongue is common.

The heart is one of the organs most active in the summer. This central muscle pumps blood and carries heat, oxygen, and nutrients throughout the body. It works closely with the lungs to gain oxygen and with the digestive system to obtain nutrients. Heart rate and rhythm are determined by the breathing and the mental and emotional state.

The heart pumps some 3,000 gallons of blood each day to the neighboring lungs, through which all blood must pass to obtain oxygen. Then the blood is returned to the heart, which pumps this nourishing breath of life to oxygenate and nourish all parts of the body.

Blood pressure is the force exerted by the blood inside the blood vessels. The pressure fluctuates as the heart beats. Factors that affect blood pressure levels are sex, age, weight, diet, activity, and stress level. Avoid stressful physical, mental, and emotional situations— as well as smoking, alcohol, and caffeine—to decrease high blood pressure. If your heart is weak or the blood vessel tone is low, then low blood pressure may exist. This most commonly occurs with young, thin women who do not exercise. Low blood pressure can cause general weakness and lethargy, lightheadedness, slow mental processes, and poor circulation. A generally good building diet will help this condition, but an active exercise program is the best remedy.

Bitter foods and herbs are considered strengthening to the heart and small intestine, though an excess of this flavor may injure them. A balance of the 5 flavors in the diet— sweet, sour, spicy, bitter, and salty—is what keeps the body in harmony. The Nei Ching offers this wisdom: "If people pay attention to the five flavors and blend them well, their bones will remain straight, their muscles will remain tender and young, breath and blood will circulate freely, the pores will be in fine texture, and consequently breath and bones will be filled with the essence of life."[3]

DIET AND NORMAL HEART FUNCTION

For the heart to remain healthy, it must always be remembered that the liver and the kidneys must be healthy too, because they are the filters of the blood which is pumped by the heart. Good general health revolves around the chemistry of proper digestion. The tremendous importance of a proper dietary regimen and the proper choice and preparation of our foods cannot be stressed enough. Foods and how they are used by our bodies are the key to overall health, as well as to normal heart function.

Improper dietary habits begin early in life and lead to saturation of the body with toxins and chemical imbalance. If the organs are not too badly damaged, as a result of this long-developing disease state, recovery certainly follows if the chemical disturbance is removed and the body cleansed. The organs can then be brought back into balance with a proper diet. Many heart problems are exacerbated by the daily use of caffeinated tea and soft drinks, coffee, tobacco, and alcoholic beverages. Lack of exercise is an important factor to consider regarding the heart's vitality. We are never too old to begin a regular exercise program that is fun and exhilarating to the spirit, as part of each day.

DIETARY GUIDELINES FROM SOME EXPERTS

1. Study the charts [chapter 9] pertaining to the importance of keeping well balanced in the chemical forces of the body (such as acid-alkaline balance and food combining).[4]

Harold J. Reilly & Ruth Brod

2. Moderation should ever be the golden rule in the diet, especially for the heart patient. A meal of many courses and heavy food throws a sudden load on the heart, which then is obliged to pump an extra supply of blood to digest it. Frequent small meals are better than overeating at any one meal or alternating between feast and famine. Sweet desserts and fatty foods, including fatty meats and gravies, should give way to vegetable soup, lean meats, vegetables, salads, and fruits.[5]

Dr. Henry Bieler

3. For better function, rest occasionally from foods.[6]

William LeSassier

4. Avoid foods that are processed, pasteurized, fried in hot oil, canned, salted, fatty foods, sugar, coffee, caffeinated tea, and alcohol.[7]

Nathan Pritikin & Leonard J. Hofer

5. Use water that is filtered, purified, distilled, or solarized, for cooking, drinking and bathing. Solarized water can be color-energized for summer in the cooling blue or green color. By leaving water in the sunlight in colored glass bottles for several days, the color vibration is transferred to the water, which then can be used as a drink to balance certain disharmonies in the body.[8]

Stanley Burroughs

6. Avoid eating dead protein foods that acidify, congest, and putrify in the body. These foods include pasteurized milk and cheese, over-cooked meats, over-cooked fish and eggs (especially the whites). Utilize fresh live foods with a minimum of processing and chemical contamination.[9]

Dr. Henry Bieler

7. Rejuvenate and strengthen the body daily with herbal tonics, teas, and seasonings in the diet. Special herbs to stimulate, purify, and vitalize the heart and blood include: hawthorn berries (heart disorders), ginseng root (stamina, virility), comfrey root (tones, clears, strengthens the intestinal mucus membrane), fennel and any seeds (gas and digestion), borage tastes like celery, the purple flowers are edible (bring happiness). Other cardiac herbs are: motherwort, asparagus, goldenseal, peppermint, pansy, sorrel, and valerian root. Cayenne pepper is very high in vitamin C and is a heart stimulant as well. It acts as a blood cleanser to help eliminate impurities. It has been used as a revival stimulant for those who have suffered from heart attacks. Hot greens like mustard greens, watercress, cauliflower, or cabbage and garlic in your diet are good for strong, clean blood.[10]

Elson M. Haas, M.D.

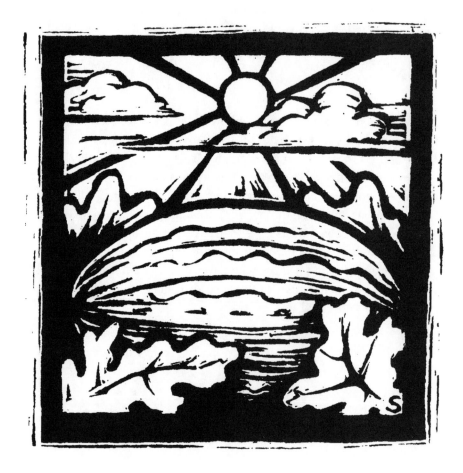

EAT MORE VEGETABLES! THE
LEAFY VARIETY WOULD BE PREFERABLE
TO THOSE OF THE POD NATURE SUCH
AS DRIED BEANS OR PEAS, OR THE LIKE.[11] [1657-002]

—EDGAR CAYCE

SUMMERTIDE FARE

BENEFICIAL SUMMER FOODS

ORGANS: Heart and small intestine

TIME: June 21 to mid-August

COLOR: Red

FRUITS: All edible local wild berries—blackberries, blueberries, gooseberries, strawberries, raspberries, elderberries, chokeberries, loganberries, mulberries, and currants; papaya, mango, pineapple, peach, apricot, and cherries (July); all melons and apples. VEGETABLES: Bitter foods and herbs; hot greens such as mustard, watercress, and collards; stronger greens such as arugula, radicchio, tango, frisee, mizuna, green oak, cocarde, dandelion leaves, and nasturtium leaves can be combined with milder greens —spinach, chard, cabbage, cauliflower, asparagus, peas, green beans, sprouted mung and lentils, and alfalfa; sea palm and nori for minerals; eggplant, artichokes, and onion to add variation. HERBS AND SEEDS: Flax, chia, garlic, ginger, cayenne, ginseng, red clover, sorrel, valerian root, hawthorn, yarrow, paprika, nettle, and rosemary. GRAINS: Oats, oat bran, corn, quinoa, and brown rice. MEAT AND DAIRY: Fish, goat's milk, and goat cheese.

FOODS TO AVOID IN SUMMER

Foods that put stress on the heart and small intestine in summer include alcohol and drugs, sugar and honey, foods with chemical additives, coffee, chocolate, and ice cream. Avoid overeating—especially meat, cheese, and eggs.

✿ CARRIE'S BERRIES WITH VANILLA YOGURT SAUCE

Fruits are a natural blood thinner for summer, adding more liquid to the diet. Plain yogurt is valued in the diet as a fermented food for its beneficial cultures. However, the cultures in yogurt are destroyed when refined sugar products are added to it. If you try to make yogurt with pasteurized milk, it will not thicken due to the hormones and antibiotics present in modern-day milk production.

INGREDIENTS	AMOUNT
organic berries	3 C.
plain organic yogurt	³/₄ C.
vanilla extract or bean seeds	1 tsp.
fresh apple juice	3 T.
ground nutmeg	¹/₄ tsp.
almonds or pine nuts (ground)	2 T.
flaxseed (ground)	1 T.

This is my recipe for keeping away from the stove and cooking pots on hot summer mornings. Take conscious advantage of the fresh fruits and vegetables of summer to build a strong body for winter!

Clean and cut the berries (if they are large) and divide between two bowls. Combine remaining ingredients and pour equal parts over berries. Sprinkle the ground nuts and seeds on top. This makes a light but hearty breakfast or snack.

✿ COLD ROSE-HIP SOUP WITH RASPBERRIES

Rose hips (the cherrylike fruit of the wild rose) are a favorite staple food in Sweden for good reason: They are 20 to 40 times higher in vitamin C than oranges, and vitamin C is a marvelous detoxifier. It neutralizes most poisons, both those produced in the body and those picked up from food or the environment. It stimulates the production of antibodies and white blood cells and inhibits the growth of practically all pathogenic bacteria and viruses.

INGREDIENTS	AMOUNT
rose hips	¹/₂ C.
water	4 C.
kuzu root powder	¹/₄ C.
apple or cherry juice	2 C.
raspberries	1 C.
lemon juice	2 T.
heavy cream or yogurt	¹/₃ C.
vanilla	1 tsp.
maple syrup (optional)	to taste

The Swedish people are known for their good health and beautiful complexions, perhaps because adequate amounts of vitamin C in their daily diet help keep collagen strong and elastic. This keeps all the tissues of the body, including the skin and muscles, healthy and smooth.

Rose hips are sold in every supermarket in Sweden and are found in most natural foods stores in the West. They are used in soups, teas, jellies, and desserts and offer optimal nutrition in a variety of interesting dishes.

Bring rose hips and water to a boil (rosehips may be ground to powder if desired). Cover and simmer for 30 minutes. Let sediment settle, then strain. Reboil and thicken with the kuzu starch thinned in cold water. Cool and add to blender with remaining ingredients; process until smooth. Garnish with a swirl of fresh cream and a mint leaf, borage flower, or viola if desired. Serves 4.

THE SOFT DRINK–FREE BODY

The artificial, oversweet flavorings of soft drinks just cannot compare to the subtle, fragrant, natural flavors found in fruits and vegetables. These are some simple ideas that will smooth the transition to the soft drink–free body.

1. If you are addicted to the caffeine in soft drinks, decrease consumption by half every other day until your body adjusts to one-fourth of your usual intake.
2. Fasting for up to 4 days on fruit or vegetable juices aids the body in the adjustment, and often the cravings for junk foods disappear as the body cleans house.
3. Do not allow soft drinks in your home. If you and your family cannot find them, they will not be consumed.
4. Keep pleasant-tasting, premade herbal tea and juice combination drinks on hand where they are easily reachable by all.
5. Plain water can be flavored with lemon, lime, and orange juice and rind—if it is organic; maple syrup may also be added for sweetness.
6. Offer thirsty individuals diluted fruit juices or vegetable juices and serve them in attractive containers, garnished for visual appeal with slices of fruit, vegetables, a whole cinnamon stick, sprinkle of nutmeg, fresh herbs, or edible flowers.
7. Make juicing a family activity. Watermelon going through the juicer attracts kids like bees to a hive. Let your children make their own juice with you there to supervise.
8. Start a tradition of juicing at family gatherings.

There are endless combinations to be discovered. Here are a few simple recipes to start off with.

✿ GINGER ALE

The ginger is great for digestion, but mainly it just tastes delicious.

Push the ginger, lemon, and grapes through the juicer. Pour the juice into a glass, add an equal amount of sparkling water, and stir in whey powder. Garnish with lemon slice.

INGREDIENTS	AMOUNT
slice of fresh gingerroot	1/4 inch
lemon	1 wedge
green grapes (with stems)	1 bunch
chilled sparkling water	as needed
whey powder	2 T.
lemon slice	garnish

✿ APPLE-MINT FIZZ

Fill a pitcher with ice, and juice directly into it. Push the mint and lemon wedge through the hopper with apple slices. Shake juice with ice to chill, and pour about 1/2 cup through a strainer into each tall glass, fill glass with sparkling water, and stir in whey powder. Garnish with strawberries and mint, if desired. Serves 4.

INGREDIENTS	AMOUNT
apples	2
fresh mint sprigs	4 to 6
lemon	1/4
chilled sparkling water	as needed
whey powder	1 T.
frozen strawberries (optional)	2 to 3

✿ BERRY-GRAPE SPRITZER

Push fruit through the juicer and mix 1 part sparkling water to 2 parts juice. Garnish with lime slices. Serves 4.

INGREDIENTS	AMOUNT
your favorite berries	2 C.
grapes (with stems)	1 bunch
lime (with peel)	1/4
sparkling water	as needed
lime slices	garnish

✿ CITRUS COOLER

Push fruit through the juicer and mix with sparkling water to taste. Garnish with lime, pineapple, or orange. Serves 4.

    Note: Use organic fruits when including the peel or skin.

INGREDIENTS	AMOUNT
pineapple (with skin)	*2 slices*
oranges (peeled with	*2*
white left intact)	
lime (with skin)	*1 wedge*
sparkling water	*as needed*
lime, pineapple, or orange	*garnish*

ROSE WATER

Step back in time and use rose water to perfume your life and flavor your food. The use of rose water in cooking is said to strengthen the brain and heart. The rose is the most superior of all scents in the floral realm. Rose works simultaneously on the physical, emotional, and spiritual bodies, purifying and uplifting all three. It has the least toxic oil of all the flowers.

SUMMER DRINK

You can make a delicious summer drink by adding 1 drop of rose oil (not rose water) to 1 gallon of water. Shake it up, and then take one drop of that liquid and add it to another fresh gallon of water. The resulting mixture is highly refreshing. This single drop still carries the power to scent the water, even though it has been diluted almost a million times. Rose oils from India and Bulgaria are considered to be the best.

CURRY

The name "curry" is thought to be derived from *kari,* a southern Indian word that refers primarily to a spicy stew. The popularity of Indian curry spread to the West during the 1800s when curry powders were carried in the ships for the servants of the East India Company. Curries are stimulating to the digestive system and the metabolism. They can be served over grains such as millet or quinoa. This praiseworthy curry is made with coconut milk, which is a healthy fat as long as it is not overheated.

✸ SAVORY GOLDEN CURRY PASTE

Toast the cumin and fenugreek in a small dry skillet until light brown. Remove outer leaf of lemongrass stalk and slice lower 6 inches; place in a blender or food processor. (If lemongrass is unavailable, add 1 tablespoon of lemon rind instead.) Finely mince the garlic and add it to the blender along with the remaining ingredients. Process the mixture until it forms a paste; cover and chill. The extra paste keeps for up to 2 weeks. Makes about ³/₄ cup.

INGREDIENTS	AMOUNT
cumin seed	1 T.
fenugreek seed	1 tsp.
lemongrass (or lemon rind)	1 stalk
garlic cloves (large)	3
onion (medium)	¹/₂
fresh gingerroot	1 T.
jalapeño chilies (seeded) (optional)	1 to 3
turmeric	¹/₄ tsp.
tamari	2 T.
lemon juice	1 tsp.

✸ MONK'S VEGETARIAN CURRY

Finely chop the mushrooms and slice the broccoli and carrot into bite-size pieces. Remove seeds from red pepper and slice 4 whole red pepper rings to reserve for garnish. Dice the remaining red pepper and set aside. In a wok or large deep skillet, heat the Curry Paste for 2 minutes and add the water or broth, vegetables, and mushrooms. Bring to a boil and turn off the heat. Add coconut milk and lemon juice and stir, then cover the curry and allow to stand for 15 minutes. Serve over basmati rice (recipe follows), millet, or quinoa, using the red pepper rings for garnish. Serves 4.

INGREDIENTS	AMOUNT
mushrooms (mixed)	3 C.
broccoli (florets)	4 C.
carrot	1
red bell pepper	1
Savory Golden Curry Paste	³/₄ C.
water or broth	¹/₂ C.
lowfat coconut milk	1¹/₂ C.
lemon juice	1¹/₂ T.
basmati rice	

❁ BASMATI RICE WITH CILANTRO

Rinse the rice and combine with water. Bring to a boil, reduce heat and simmer (covered) until tender (20–30 minutes). Allow to cool for 10 minutes, then add the sesame oil and finely chopped cilantro leaves. Toss to incorporate. Serve a vegetable curry over the rice. A mixed green salad is good for a cooling effect and especially tasty with Pine Nut Dressing (below). Serves 4 to 6.

INGREDIENTS	AMOUNT
basmati rice	2 C.
pure water	4 C.
sesame oil	1 T.
fresh cilantro	1 C.

❁ PINE NUT SALAD DRESSING

Place ingredients in blender and process until creamy, or whisk the ingredients together, leaving the pine nuts whole. Makes ³/₄ cup.

INGREDIENTS	AMOUNT
white wine	3 T.
Dijon or stone-ground mustard	2 tsp.
dried thyme	1 tsp.
dried oregano	¹/₄ tsp.
cold-pressed olive oil	4 T.
flaxseed oil	2 T.
pine nuts	4 T.

❁ FRESH TUNA SALADE NIÇOISE

This delicious salad is a real summer treat, a complete protein meal providing omega-3 fatty acids, vitamins, and minerals. This dish is particularly memorable shared with friends for a special occasion. I first made this recipe while on a long sail in the South Pacific.

In a blender, puree until smooth the garlic, capers, anchovies, 2 tablespoons of parsley, and olives. Gradually add ¹/₄ cup olive oil, blend well. Reserve this olive paste for garnish on tuna. In a separate bowl or jar with a lid, combine the lemon juice, vinegar, shallots, and red pepper with ²/₃ cup olive oil. (The recipe can be prepared to this point one day ahead. Cover and chill mixtures separately.)

Steam the green beans until crisp-tender, about 5 minutes; refresh under

cold running water, drain, and add to
the bowl with the vinaigrette. Toss
well, then let marinate 1 to 2 hours.
Combine the remaining 2 tablespoons
of olive oil with the tamari and marinate tuna as above.

Steam new potatoes until tender;
drain and cool slightly. Slice potatoes
1/4-inch thick; cover and set aside.

Place the tuna steaks in a broiling
pan and rub with the olive oil and
tamari mixture. Season lightly with
red pepper and broil to desired ten-
derness. Cool slightly, then slice across
the grain, 1/3-inch thick. Set aside.
Remove the green beans from the
vinaigrette, then add mixed greens to
vinaigrette and toss well to coat.

INGREDIENTS	AMOUNT
garlic cloves (large)	2
capers (drained)	1 1/2 T.
anchovy fillets (drained)	1/4 C.
chopped flat-leaf parsley (divided)	4 T.
Kalamata olives (pitted)	1 C.
virgin olive oil (divided)	1 C.
fresh lemon juice	2 T.
apple cider vinegar	2 T.
small shallots or scallions	8
red pepper	1/8 tsp.
green beans	1 lb.
tamari	1 1/2 T.
fresh tuna steak, about 1 inch thick (cut into equal chunks)	1 1/4 lb.
new potatoes	1 lb. or 12 small
mixed greens (bite-size pieces)	8 C.
ripe tomatoes (sliced 1/4 inch thick)	2

To serve, arrange the tuna slices,
tomato slices, and potato slices
around the rims of 6 serving plates.
Mound the tossed greens in the center and top with the marinated beans. Top
each slice of tuna with 1/2 teaspoon of the reserved olive paste. Garnish with
chopped parsley. Serves 6.

✿ BABY SPINACH SALAD WITH CURRANTS

Dark leafy green salads are excellent
summer blood builders due to high
chlorophyll content. For variation,
add mixed lettuces to the spinach or
red chard for color. Currants are a
type of miniature raisin from the
Corinth grape. They are a storehouse
of minerals, with an abundant supply
of potassium, phosphorus, magnesium, iron, and calcium, and also vit-

INGREDIENTS	AMOUNT
baby spinach and mixed greens	6 C.
Spike Shake (p. 41)	to season
avocado (sliced)	1 sliced
tomatoes, vine ripened (sliced)	2 sliced
currants	1/2 C.
scallions	1/3 C.
sunflower seeds	1 C.

amins A, B complex, and a trace of C. Currants are high in carbohydrates and have some protein and little fat. Sunflower seeds contain complete protein—a handful is equal to the protein in an average-size steak. Avocados contain many enzymes for good digestion.

Wash the greens well, dry, and tear into bite-size pieces. Place them on a serving plate and season with Spike Shake. Arrange avocado and tomato over the greens. Sprinkle the currants, scallions, and sunflower seeds over the top. This salad is good with the Pine Nut Dressing (p. 77). Serves 4.

✿ GREEN GODDESS DRESSING

Creamy goat cheese is often easy to digest for those with sensitivity to cheese made with cow's milk. Its high buffering capacity makes it useful for calming and healing stomach ulcers. This delightful soft green dressing should be made with fresh herbs.

Place all ingredients in a blender and process until creamy. Serve this dressing over any mixture of greens and vegetables you wish. It is particularly good with mâche and miners lettuce. Makes about ¹/₂ cup.

INGREDIENTS	AMOUNT
creamy goat cheese or feta cheese	2 T.
cold-pressed olive oil	2 T.
flaxseed oil or hempseed oil	1 T.
fresh lemon juice	2 T.
apple juice	1 T.
fresh rosemary	1 T.
fresh chives (chopped)	2 T.
tamari	1 T.
maple syrup (optional)	1 tsp.

✿ SMOKE AND THUNDER PEPPER POLENTA

Polenta originates from the simple staple dish of the ancient Roman legions called *puls* or *pulementum*. It was a mush made of millet or spelt, the common grains of the time until the arrival of corn from the New World in the sixteenth century. Today yellow, white, red, or blue cornmeal is used in fine, medium, or coarse grinds to create versatile, soothing, and memorable dishes. Cornmeal is best when freshly ground; old cornmeal has poor absorption qualities and often has a bitter taste. This recipe is my idea of a real Southwestern feast. I keep a jar of roasted red peppers on hand for convenience. Serve this with a simple chili sauce.

In a heavy saucepan with a thick bottom, place the liquids and a handful of the finely ground yellow cornmeal; bring to a boil and add the paprika. Lower the heat to a slow simmer and add the remaining cornmeal, stirring well after each addition. Continue to stir around the sides and bottom and cook enough to thicken, at least 20 minutes, or enough to support the weight of the spoon. Add the red pepper, onion, tamari, butter, and cheese; stir until combined. Cover and allow to stand for 5 minutes. Serve the polenta hot by the spoonful or pour it into a parchment-lined sheet pan or loaf pan, smooth the top, and refrigerate. Once the polenta has firmed, it can be cut into slices or shaped with cookie cutters into stars, moons, or triangles and baked to reheat. Garnish with whole dry chili peppers, chives, or crumbled goat feta, and serve with salad greens. I like to serve the polenta with a green side salad. Smoke and Thunder Pepper Polenta is served with the following Basic Red Chili Sauce for dipping. Fresh orange wedges are the perfect cooling complement for this dish. Serves 5 or 6.

INGREDIENTS	AMOUNT
water or stock	4 C.
sherry or Madeira wine	1/4 C.
yellow cornmeal (finely ground)	1 C.
paprika	2 T.
yellow cornmeal (coarsely ground)	1 C.
roasted red pepper (chopped)	1/2 C.
green onion or chives (chopped)	1/2 C.
tamari	1 1/2 tsp.
butter (organic) or cream	2 T.
feta cheese (crumbled)	1/3 C.
whole dry chilies	for garnish
chives (chopped)	for garnish
mixed salad greens (optional)	
Red Chili Sauce (recipe follows)	
oranges, cut in wedges	6

✿ BASIC RED CHILI SAUCE

This simple chili sauce is the perfect accompaniment to the smoke and thunder taste of the polenta. Serve the sauce in tiny dipping bowls arranged next to the polenta, so that each person can sample the spicy flavor. Chili peppers of all kinds benefit the heart and circulation. Hot peppers are a stimulating herb that helps prevent heart attack, strokes, colds, flu,

INGREDIENTS	AMOUNT
brown rice flour	4 tsp.
water or stock	2 C.
red chili powder	1/4 C.
garlic (minced)	1 tsp.
oregano	1 tsp.
Worcestershire sauce or tamari	1 tsp.
olive oil, butter, or cream	2 T.

diminished vitality, headaches, indigestion, depression, and arthritis.

Heat a small iron skillet and dry roast the brown rice flour until lightly toasted. Stir in $\frac{1}{4}$ cup stock and add the chili powder; cook for 1 minute. Gradually add the remaining stock, stirring constantly to prevent lumps. Simmer on low heat for 10 to 15 minutes; remove from heat and add the remaining ingredients. Cover tightly and allow flavors to meld before serving (about 20 minutes). Chili sauce keeps well and can be made in advance.

PASTA PARADOX

Like white bread, white pasta is a staple food in many regions. Experience has taught us that white breads do not support health, and this is true also of white pasta. The use of fresh whole grain breads and pastas is a key factor in maintaining a healthy body.

The advantage of using whole grain products was shown during World War I, when shortages caused the Danish government to forbid the milling of grains. Nutrition in Denmark was so improved during the war years that the death rate fell 34 percent. The incidence of cancer, diabetes, high blood pressure, and heart and kidney diseases dropped markedly, and evidences of positive health greatly increased. Much the same improvement occurred in England during and after World War II, when grains were only slightly milled.

Today we have a colorful, nutritious variety of whole grain pastas to choose from, and many of these are organic. I will begin with my favorites: the delicious and addicting Soba noodle—60 percent whole wheat flour and 40 percent buckwheat flour; Udon—100 percent whole wheat flour; spinach, red pepper, and veggie spirals—90 percent whole wheat. There are wheat-free pastas also, such as corn, quinoa, and sesame, to complement the richness and variety of seasonal sauces and toppings.

The freshest pastas are made at home. Grind the whole, organic grains yourself, using a grain mill. A grain mill, preferably a good manual one (for when the electricity goes out), is a valuable tool for making fresh whole grain flours and cornmeal for every culinary use.

The oils in flour and flour products usually become rancid seven to ten days after the grain is broken down or milled. Grain products and flour are best stored in the refrigerator or freezer to extend shelf life.

✿ SPIRAL PASTA WITH CHERRY TOMATOES AND SWEET BASIL

This is a longtime favorite summer pasta dish that serves equally well for lunch or dinner. It is simple to prepare, with a fresh and light flavor for summer. Fresh basil must be used in this recipe for best results. Always choose whole grain pastas over white pasta. This pasta is good served with the Bitter Summer Greens Salad (p. 83).

INGREDIENTS	AMOUNT
whole grain pasta spirals	4 C.
fresh basil leaves	1 C.
cherry tomatoes (halved)	35 to 40
mayonnaise	$^{1}/_{2}$ C.
paprika	$^{1}/_{4}$ tsp.
oregano	1 tsp.
marjoram	1 tsp.
apple juice (or cider vinegar or lemon juice)	1 T.

Boil enough water to cover the pasta and cook until tender (about 5 minutes); drain, refresh with cold water, then set aside to cool. Chop the basil leaves leaving 5 whole leaves for garnish. Add half of the cherry tomatoes and half of the chopped basil to the pasta and toss. Place the remaining half of the cherry tomatoes in a blender with all the remaining ingredients. Process until creamy, then combine with the pasta. Garnish with a whole cherry tomato and a whole fresh basil leaf. Serves 5.

❁ FAVORITE BASIL PESTO

Pestos are herb pastes that can be made in endless variety. They add new flavor to vegetable, grain, dairy, and meat dishes and keep for 3 or 4 weeks in the refrigerator. Whenever olive oil is used in an uncooked recipe, such as pesto, consider replacing a portion of the olive oil with hempseed oil to get your omega-3 and -6 essential fatty acids. I always use cayenne pepper in place of black pepper in all recipes. The particles of

INGREDIENTS	AMOUNT
fresh basil leaves	2 C.
garlic cloves (large)	2
freshly grated Parmesan cheese	$^{1}/_{2}$ C.
pecorino Romano cheese	2 T.
pine nuts or walnuts	$^{1}/_{4}$ C.
cold-pressed olive oil	$^{1}/_{3}$ C.
hempseed oil	2 T.
cayenne pepper	to taste
sea salt	to taste

cracked black peppercorns are said to irritate the liver four times more than alcohol. Whole black peppercorns can be used to flavor a dish and then removed.

A food processor with an **S** blade makes making pesto easy. Process the basil, garlic, cheeses, and nuts. With the machine running, add the oils slowly and season to taste. If you are making pesto with a blender, put the oil in first. With the machine running, add the basil and garlic (through the blender-top hole). Then add the nuts and cheese. Season to taste. Store pesto in the refrigerator with a thin coating of oil or water on top to keep air out. Cover the container tightly. Makes about 1 cup.

✿ PESTO ROUNDS

These simple pesto rounds are great as an elegant appetizer or alongside a fresh salad as a meal. There are many variations of goat cheese and pesto—along with nuts, seeds, and herbs that garnish the top—with which to experiment throughout the seasons to make a festive display.

INGREDIENTS	AMOUNT
cucumber rounds	12
creamy goat cheese	1/4 C.
Basil or Rosemary Pesto (pp. 82, 167)	1/3 C.
sunflower seeds or pine nuts	1/4 C.

Cover each cucumber round with cheese, leaving edges of cucumber to show. Spread the pesto over the cheese, leaving edges of cheese to show the layered colors. Sprinkle each cucumber with fresh-shelled sunflower seeds or pine nuts. Serves 4.

✿ BITTER SUMMER GREENS SALAD WITH FRESH CORN

Bitter summer greens such as those used here help to stimulate the heart energy and purify the blood. Do not let the term "bitter" scare you! This is a delicious and simple summer salad.

Wash and separate the frisee and arugula lettuces, shake or spin dry, and blot with paper towels. Remove the outer leaves of the endive, quarter the heart lengthwise and separate the leaves. Put the lettuces into a clean glass bowl. Crush the garlic cloves and combine with oil, vinegar, and seasonings. Add the dressing to the bowl containing the lettuces, and cover with a large plate. Shake it until the dressing evenly coats the lettuce. Arrange lettuces on a serving plate; husk the corn and cut away the kernels, sprinkling the fresh corn over the top. Serves 5.

INGREDIENTS	AMOUNT
frisee lettuce	1 head
arugula lettuce	1 head
Belgian endive	1 head
garlic cloves	1 or 2
cold-pressed olive oil	1/4 C.
apple cider vinegar	1 T.
cayenne pepper	1 pinch
tamari	1 tsp.
fresh raw corn	1 ear

✿ SUMMER SOLSTICE SORBET

A common mistake made in the flame of summer is eating ice cream, which is rich and heats the blood more than any other food. In healing, ice cream is recommended as a winter food, and only if it is fresh and of good quality. Another common mistake—

INGREDIENTS	AMOUNT
lemongrass stalks or lemon rind (organic)	3
pure water or lemon verbena tea	$3^1/_4$ C.
fresh mint leaves	$^1/_2$ C. ($^1/_4$ C. dry)
vanilla extract	$^1/_2$ tsp.
honey	2 T.
light coconut milk	$^3/_4$ C.

in any season—is drinking ice water, which shocks the warm stomach tissue. The various fruit and herb sorbets will bridge the gap nicely between rich ice cream and ice water. They melt in your mouth and are clean and refreshing. The lemongrass used in this unique recipe is wonderful in many dishes, if you can get it in your area. If you substitute lemon peel for lemongrass, replace the water with lemon verbena tea.

Discard outer leaves and trim root ends of the lemongrass stalks; slice stalks up to the dried thin upper portion. If using lemons, peel the rind off with a knife. In a saucepan, simmer the lemongrass or lemon rind with the water, cover for 5 minutes. Bruise the mint leaves to release the natural oils. Remove pan from the heat, add mint, and cover. Let stand 20 minutes, then stir in the remaining ingredients. In a blender, puree mixture, then strain through a fine sieve into a bowl—pressing hard on the solids. Freeze in ice-cream maker or ice cube trays. To refresh the sorbet from the freezer, let stand for 10 minutes and then crush the cubes in a blender. Garnish with fresh mint, or sprinkle with powdered sugar or fresh fruit. Makes 3 cups.

LATE SUMMER RESTORATION

LATE SUMMER

The end of summer is considered a season by itself in the Five Element Theory. This period of time has aspects of all the seasons—such as hot and cold—or sometimes other extremes occur during the transitional period between summer and autumn, from mid-August through September 22.

Late summer is correlated with the element Earth, which relates to the cycles in Nature and is central to all the other elements. The center is the direction associated with the Earth element. The **spleen**, **stomach**, and Earth element rule the center, which relates to the four corners of the Earth, the four directions. The Earth element plays an important role during transitional times and seasonal changes. During these times, it is most important to stay centered.

The stomach and the spleen work together to digest the foods we eat and distribute the resulting energy throughout the body. Proper functioning of these organs is vital for prevention of illness. Healthy eating habits play the key role in keeping digestion working efficiently and maintaining a strong stomach and spleen.

THE STOMACH

The digestive organs and their functioning reflect the influence of diet, mental activity, and emotions. In fact, the stomach is one of the most sensitive organs in the body. The whole digestive system is finely tuned by the nervous system, so stress of any kind affects its function; the state of the emotions is closely linked to eating habits and the ability to process food. Taking care with the diet, chewing well, taking your time, and not overeating, are important. Choose a relaxed setting away from chemical pollutants, and do not eat too many different kinds of food at one time. Too much or too frequent eating will overwork, weaken, and even wear out the digestive system to the point that it breaks down to receive the rest it needs.

After a meal, it is beneficial to enjoy a short spell of relaxation. Then the body needs to move to aid digestion and to assimilate and distribute the nutrients. The way your body is processing your food can be judged by your moment-to-moment state of energy. All foods eaten at the same time must be broken down to the same consistency before the stomach will actually begin to empty. There are different digestive substances that break down each kind of food; fats and proteins take longer to digest than do carbohydrates. Simple fruits may take 10 to 20 minutes, while meats might take 45 to 90 minutes— depending on how well they are chewed. If fruit is eaten at the same time as meat, the fruit will have to stay an extra hour in the stomach. During this time, fermentation will take place, introducing gas into the system and causing indigestion, belching, or cramps.

A simple list of foods in order of decreasing ease of digestibility and increasing length of time in the stomach includes: fruits, vegetables, grains, beans, seeds, nuts, dairy products, and meats. To better understand the basic art of balancing your diet, consult the Wisdom Chart on food combining in chapter 9.

❀ STRAWBERRY AND BANANA FAST

The strawberry and banana fast is a very agreeable way to cleanse the stomach; it should be practiced by those who have difficulty in digesting protein and fat. Choose organic fruit whenever possible. Before taking these foods, clear the digestive tract with the Epsom Salts or Castor Oil internal bath in chapter 7.

INGREDIENTS (per drink)	AMOUNT
organic bananas	1 C.
organic strawberries	½ C.
vanilla	scant ⅛ tsp.
pure water	¼ C.

TIME: Late Summer
TIME FRAME: 1 to 3 Days

Clean, cut, peel, and combine the above and blend to a creamy consistency. This drink is taken whenever you are hungry. Whole bananas and strawberries can be eaten as desired throughout your fast, but no other food is added except pure water and herbal tea. Remember to skin brush (chapter 7) each day while fasting. Break the fast with a combination of the following healing foods.

HEALING STOMACH FOODS

Our stomachs benefit from simply eating the super foods that are healing to this important organ. These are good foods to break your fast and to use for stomach distress, sick stomach, stomach pain, and stomach ulcers.

1. Aloe vera juice and papaya puree (combined)
2. Carrot juice and carrot puree
3. Coconut milk
4. Goat's milk
5. Sweet potato
6. Parsnip
7. Flaxseed tea
8. Slippery elm tea
9. Raw cabbage juice

✿ STOMACH ULCER DIET

In Europe, there are health resorts that specialize in treating stomach ulcers. This specific diet is followed for 1 week. Afterward, a diet with emphasis on food combining and healing stomach foods should be eaten. Citrus foods and all aluminum pots, pans, and foil should be avoided.

TIME: Late Summer
TIME FRAME: 7 days

DAYS 1 THROUGH 3: Eat carrots only: juiced, steamed, raw, pureed, grilled, or baked. Have a combination of these. Flaxseed tea and slippery elm tea may also be added, 1 cup per day if desired. Pepsin tablets may be added also. Comfrey and pepsin herbal capsules work in the stomach to help heal ulcers, soothe the digestive tract, and dissolve mucus from the walls of the intestines.

DAYS 4 THROUGH 7: Morning: Carrot juice or carrot soup
Midmorning: Potato juice or potato broth
Noon: Potato and carrot (as above)
Midafternoon: Herbal tea with cream
Evening: Carrot and baked potato
Bedtime: Herbal tea and cream

New therapies for stomach ulcers offer treatment for the disease. However, if you have a tendency toward ulcers and stomach weakness, a protective diet and occasional fast are very beneficial.

RAW CABBAGE JUICE

Raw cabbage juice has germicidal properties. It is known to sooth stomach ulcers with its vitamin U. The juice can be mixed with honey for coughing and hoarseness. Cabbage glutamine has been used to treat alcoholism, anemia, fatigue, infections, intestinal parasites, stones, and arthritis.[13]

THE SPLEEN AND PANCREAS

The spleen is a central organ, both physiologically and anatomically. Defects in spleen energy can affect the whole body because the spleen distributes the energy obtained from foods throughout the body. The other organs depend on this distribution of energy for life. In the present day, it is quite common for the spleen to be diseased because we eat too many sweet foods.

The spleen consists of lymphatic tissue and produces plasma cells, which make antibodies, and is part of the immune system's defense against disease. It stores blood and destroys old blood cells, and is the reserve organ for blood formation in the adult. In the fetus, it is an important organ for blood formation, especially red blood cells.

The pancreas is associated with the spleen, secreting hormones into the blood. Insulin, the main pancreatic hormone, lowers the blood sugar level by stimulating glucose use by the cells; the pancreas also secretes the hormone glucagon to raise the blood sugar level. Another important function of the pancreas is the secretion of pancreatic enzymes directly into the small intestine, assisting in the digestion of fats, proteins, and carbohydrates.

The flavor of sweetness stimulates the spleen and pancreas, but too much sweet food can injure these organs. Overwork of the system can weaken the pancreas, leading to weak insulin response. The inability to clear and use up the sugar in the blood leads to "high blood sugar" (diabetes). An overresponse of the pancreas from sugar and food intake, releasing too much insulin, is called "low blood sugar" (hypoglycemia).

Countless examples show that the introduction of refined sugar into a culture's diet is accompanied by a rapid increase in infectious diseases and diabetes. The brain cells are the most sensitive to changes in blood sugar levels, resulting in mental imbalance such as depression, anxiety, and irritability. Modern use of refined sugar has brought tooth decay and mental and physical degeneration to the human race due to the destructive, concentrated, crystallized acids contained in it. Historical research shows us that, since refined sugar foods have been in wide use, physical degeneration has developed in a way that was definitely observable in a single generation. The only way to prevent further damage now, and for future generations, is to avoid overuse of cane and beet sugars in all their forms and guises.

Medically, the mental and physical degeneration can be attributed to the role of refined sugar in the depletion of many of the body's important nutrients such as protein, vitamin B, zinc, chromium, and manganese. All of these are essential for stable mental and emotional functioning; their deficiency has been associated with depression, fatigue, and low blood sugar. The Chinese healing system correlates the health of the spleen and menstrual regularity. Elimination of refined sugar in the diet may help to remedy menstrual problems such as irregularity, pain, and either insufficient or excessive bleeding.

The body makes its own sugar—human glucose, the fuel on which the body runs—from the foods we eat. These foods can be converted to glucose to run the body. There is also a reverse process when glucose is converted back to glycogen and stored in the liver, to amino acids for muscle storage, or to fatty acids and into fatty tissue. An overuse (abuse) of sugar will produce mainly fat, first deposited in the most inactive areas, especially the abdomen, thighs, and buttocks; and then, with chronic excess, stored in the internal organs—the blood vessels, heart, and kidneys. Conversely, a low sugar intake allows the body to change excess fats to glucose for ready use. Then the body is able to decongest, retexture, and finely shape itself.

HERBAL HEALERS FOR LATE SUMMER

"Native American medicine is really the traditional American medicine and is very closely linked to Chinese medicine. They both use herbal treatment in the context of an understanding of Heaven and Earth as a means of maintaining health,"[14] writes Elson M. Haas, M.D. in his book *Staying Healthy with the Seasons*. The human species has always utilized plants for healing, and present-day pharmaceutical medicine extracts the active ingredients of herbs and plants to synthesize similar drugs with stronger effects. In this respect, the metamorphosis of our use of these gifts of Nature continues. However, the use of herbs, not pharmaceuticals, for healing has long been known as the art of "simpling." Anyone can enjoy the simple pleasures of the following herbal recipes and receive traditional healing results from potent medicinal plants.

✿ ORANGE ROSEMARY TEA

Make a mild tea from these ingredients for weak stomach acidity and to stimulate hydrochloric acid for better digestion.

INGREDIENTS	AMOUNT
pure water	2 C.
dried rosemary	1 T. (2 T. if fresh)
fresh or dried orange peel (organic)	2 or 3 pieces
fresh or dried juniper berries (optional)	1 T.

In a glass or stainless-steel vessel, bring water to a boil. Remove from the heat and add the ingredients. Cover tightly and steep for 15 to 20 minutes. Drink ¹/₂ cup about ¹/₂ hour before meals. For weak digestion, avoid cold foods and do not drink anything with your meals. Bitter foods such as endive, dandelion greens, and chicory are also known to strengthen digestion.

✿ SPICE TEA

Spice tea is good to drink after a meal to relieve indigestion, hyper-acidity, or gas.

INGREDIENTS	AMOUNT
pure water	2 C.
anise, cardamom, caraway, fennel,	3 T.
or fenugreek seed	

In a glass or stainless-steel vessel, boil the water. Add 1 or more of the seeds to total 3 tablespoons. Simmer in a covered pot for 15 minutes; remove from the heat and allow to stand for another 15 minutes.

Strain and drink ¹/₂ to 1 cup after meals. Fennel or anise seed can also be chewed as an after-meal digestive aid.

✿ LICORICE MINT TEA

This is a nice calming, after-dinner tea that works as a mild laxative as well.

INGREDIENTS	AMOUNT
pure water	3 C.
licorice root	1 T.
fenugreek seed	1 T.
peppermint leaves (dried)	3 T.

In a glass or stainless-steel vessel, boil the water. Add the licorice and fenugreek. Cover and simmer for 15 minutes. Remove from the heat and add the peppermint. Cover and allow to steep another 15 minutes. Strain and enjoy.

✿ GREEN JUICE FAST

TIME: Late Summer
TIME FRAME: 1 to 3 days

For the health of the spleen, to build immunity, to energize and heal, and to calm the nerves, try this fresh juice cleanse.

Juice equal parts: romaine lettuce, celery, and parsley
$^1/_2$ part fresh comfrey leaf (optional)

Combine with an equal or lesser amount of pure water and drink immediately after juicing. Drink an 8-ounce glassful every 3 hours. In between green juice, drink Licorice Mint Tea and water.

Optional: niacin (100 mg) 2 or 3 times a day in conjunction with sweat baths, followed by a cool shower
flaxseed oil (1 teaspoon in gelatin capsules) 2 or 3 times a day with juice or tea
skin brushing daily before dressing or bathing

Important Note: Clear the digestive tract each day with a laxative herbal tea or clear the large intestine daily with enema therapy while undergoing any juice fast. If the urge for solid food is overwhelming at first, eat apples or grapes between the juice drinks until the body adjusts.

TURKISH WATERMELON FAST

These two fasts for kidney ailments have been handed down by Hannah Kroeger, who was born in Turkey and studied natural healing under the Oriental and European methods. In the Chinese system, these kidney programs would be focused upon in winter, because the kidneys deal with water in the system and, therefore, are associated with winter. However, this is a watermelon-based program and watermelons are generally only available in summer.

The watermelon is said to have originated in Africa and appears to have been introduced to the Americas by Europeans in the seventeenth century. However, M. R. Gilmore has traced some varieties of watermelon originating in North America. Among the Hopi Indians, the watermelon was sometimes a staple food. This tribe told the ethnobotanist A. F. Whiting in the 1930s that they regretted having traded their "old type" melons, which kept until February, for newer varieties that were better flavored but did not keep as well.[15] With this information, it appears that a watermelon fast is perfectly suited for the body in winter, provided that one finds the appropriate watermelon. Whole watermelon seeds are also available through herbalists, and may be used for watermelon seed tea in winter.

The Turks fast on delicious watermelon once a year. Going on watermelon for 3 to 5 days is a wonderful kidney cleanser, working as an eliminant and diuretic. It helps to eliminate debris in the large intestine and the extra water picks up toxic materials and carries them off. If you fast on watermelon, be sure to save the seeds to make watermelon seed tea for the second recipe given.

✿ WATERMELON CLEANSE FAST #1
TIME: Late Summer
TIME FRAME: 3 to 5 days

One small or medium organic watermelon for each day you will fast. If a large melon is used, $1/2$ per day is the general amount needed. Before cutting the melon, soak it first in a gallon of water and $1/2$ teaspoon Clorox bleach for 15 to 20 minutes, rinse and soak in plain water for 10 to 15 minutes and let dry. This step will purify the melon and guard against bacterial contamination. Enjoy the watermelon whenever you are hungry or thirsty. Eat only the watermelon and watermelon juice for 3 to 5 days. Once a day, in the morning or night, take a laxative herbal tea or enema therapy. Skin brush before you dress or bathe (chapter 7).

✿ WATERMELON CLEANSE FAST #2
TIME: Late Summer
TIME FRAME: 3 to 14 days

I have used this diet many times and every time the result was immediate and astounding. It balances the fluids in the system by releasing electrical currents and reestablishing the yin-yang function of the kidneys. Instructions follow this recipe.

✿ WATERMELON SEED TEA
Watermelon seeds contain glutathione, a natural antioxidant. Glutathione helps protect almost every part of the body from oxidative damage, including the eyes, lungs, and liver. It

INGREDIENTS	AMOUNT
watermelon seeds (crushed)	1 C.
pure water	3 qts.

works like the antioxidant vitamins C, E, and beta-carotene. Glutathione can be manufactured in the body from certain amino acids, but various illnesses and aging may cause a deficiency. Nutritionists suggest that you supplement your diet with natural sources of glutathione, such as watermelon seed, to give you the best cellular protection.

Boil the crushed seeds in the water for about 3 minutes. Cool, strain, and store 2 quarts in the refrigerator to keep it fresh until needed. When the first quart has reached room temperature or is lukewarm, take $1/3$ cup every hour.

> BREAKFAST: Eat watermelon.
>
> LUNCH: Plain yogurt, raw vegetables, some fish or egg yolk or rye bread (no oils).
>
> DINNER: Stewed pears or applesauce with plain yogurt or soy milk, as much as you like.

Do this diet for 3 days but continue taking the watermelon seed tea and watermelon breakfasts for 14 days total.

✿ HOMEMADE CALCIUM SUPPLEMENT

Here is a simple calcium supplement that can be used while fasting in any season or as an addition to the daily diet.

Place whole eggs in a glass jar. Cover the eggs with the fresh lemon juice.

INGREDIENTS	AMOUNT
whole eggs (from chickens without antibiotics or hormones)	3
fresh lemon juice (or enough to cover eggs)	2 C.

Put the lid on the jar and refrigerate for 24 to 36 hours. Gently agitate the jar several times during those hours. The egg shells will become paper thin. When the time has passed, carefully remove the whole eggs from the lemon juice and discard them. The lemon juice should be taken every morning for 1 month, $1/4$ to $1/2$ teaspoon to build calcium. Do this twice a year.

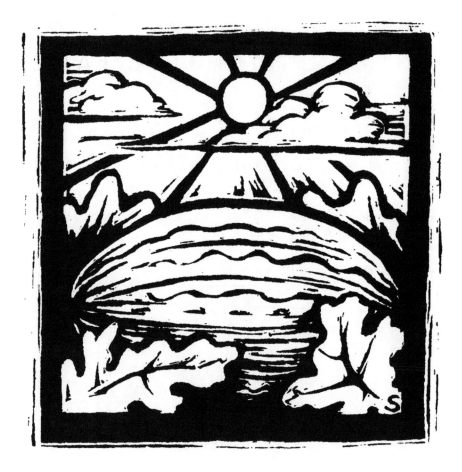

THE SEEDS WITHIN US AND THAT WHICH
BROUGHT US LIVING IS AN ANCIENT
BREATH.[16]

—PETER BLUE CLOUD

LATE SUMMERTIDE FARE

BENEFICIAL LATE SUMMER FOODS

ORGANS: Spleen, pancreas, stomach
TIME: September to late October
COLOR: Yellow
FRUITS: Local sweet fruits such as watermelon, pears, and apples; and bananas. VEG-
ETABLES AND HERBS: Sweet round, compact vegetables such as turnip, cabbage, onion,
rutabaga, and pumpkin. Sea vegetables such as arame and kombu (good in miso soup).
Peas, fennel, parsley, horseradish, and watercress. GRAINS: Millet. DAIRY: Yogurt (plain
organic)—flavor with vanilla extract, nutmeg, or cinnamon. NUTS: Walnuts, which are
harvested in September. Keep all nuts in their shells until needed. The delicate oils in nuts
become rancid soon after the shells are removed.

FOODS TO AVOID IN LATE SUMMER

Foods that stress the spleen, stomach, and pancreas in late summer include high-fat foods,
tropical fruit juices, sugar, and food additives such as MSG.

❁ BANANA ALMOND MILK

Nut milks are good alternatives to
using dairy products. I like to use
almonds for their alkaline properties. They help to neutralize excess
acids in the stomach and supply
high quality protein and calcium.
Bananas are a good source of energy and help maintain healthy skin

INGREDIENTS	AMOUNT
organic raw almonds	1/3 C.
pure water	4 C.
flaxseed	1 T.
almond butter	2 T.
honey or maple syrup	2 T.
ripe banana	1/2 C.
vanilla extract	1 tsp.

and hair. They should be eaten when ripe, with the skin speckled with dark spots.

If using whole almonds, soak them in the water overnight. In a blender, grind the flaxseed to a powder and add remaining ingredients. Process to a creamy consistency. This drink is nice sprinkled with a bit of nutmeg if desired.

✿ RED MISO DRESSING

Miso is a form of fermented soy-bean paste that is used in Japanese cuisine as a delicious stock for soups. I find that the flavor and consistency of the various kinds of miso are perfect for salad dressings. Miso is an important food to keep in your diet for the valuable minerals and beneficial bacteria that aid digestion and detoxify the intestines.

INGREDIENTS	AMOUNT
virgin olive oil	1/3 C.
tamari	1 T.
cider vinegar	2 T.
cumin, marjoram, mint, oregano, sage, tarragon, and turmeric	1 tsp. each
canola oil	1/4 C.
red miso paste	1 T.

Combine all of the ingredients except for the canola oil and miso. Use the canola oil to thin down the thick red miso paste before adding it to the finished dressing. This will keep for weeks refrigerated. Makes about 3/4 cup.

✿ ZUCCHINI BOAT SALAD

Zucchini is a great supplier of the organic sodium that our bodies need each day to nourish the adrenal glands. Zucchini boats make a quick and satisfying salad that can be a main course. Add a side dish such as Green Masala String Beans (recipe follows) and your guests will be delighted.

INGREDIENTS	AMOUNT
green and yellow zucchini (medium)	4
Red Miso Dressing (above)	1/2 C.
goat or Swiss cheese	1/2 C.
Spike Shake (p. 41)	to season
mixed dark leafy salad greens	1 lb.

Wash the zucchini and cut each one in half lengthwise. Place the zucchini in a shallow pan or on a small cookie sheet with the skin side down. Brush each piece with Red Miso Dressing and sprinkle lightly with the cheese. Top with a dash of seasoning or your choice of herbs. Bake at 325 degrees until tender (about 10 minutes). Wash and dry the salad greens and arrange on individual plates. Season the greens with Spike Shake and Red Miso Dressing. Place the warm zucchini boats on top of the greens and serve. Serves 4.

GARAM MASALA STRING BEANS

String beans are rich in chloro-phyll, which is beneficial for all tissue repair. Chlorophyll helps to neutralize some of the pollution that we eat and breathe, and helps to keep calcium and other minerals in the body.

INGREDIENTS	AMOUNT
snap beans	1 lb.
olive oil	2 T.
butter	1 tsp.
cider vinegar	1/2 tsp.
prepared mustard	2 tsp.
prepared horseradish	1 tsp.
garam masala or Curry Paste (p. 76)	1 1/2 tsp.
white miso paste or apple juice	2 tsp.
red onion (chopped)	1/2 C.

Wash and trim the beans and cut them into 1-inch pieces; steam for 3 minutes, drain. Combine all remaining ingredi-ents in order given, except for red onion. Toss in the beans and stir over low heat until the beans are coated evenly with the sauce; add red onion. Serves 4.

OPERA SALAD WITH CAPERS

This unique salad, made with crunchy raw celery and steamed carrots is served warm, tossed with Kumari Curry Dressing. It is elegant enough to be served as a main course or as a colorful side dish on a plate with fish or pasta.

INGREDIENTS	AMOUNT
carrots	4 or 5
celery stalks	3
green onion or chives	1/3 C.
capers	1 T.
Kumari Curry Dressing (p. 42)	1/3 C.
mixed salad greens	8 C.
Spike Shake (p. 41)	optional
bean sprouts (chopped)	optional

Wash all vegetables. Cut the carrots into 1 1/2-inch pieces on an angle (do not peel). Steam the carrots until tender (10–15 min-utes). Dice the celery and onion, add the capers. When the carrots are done, combine them with the celery mixture and toss with dressing. Serve over the mixed greens, seasoned with Spike Shake if desired. This salad is also good with bean sprouts added. Add them to the vegetable mixture if desired, or garnish the salad with sprouts. Serves 4.

❀ BIG SCENE SALSA AND BEAN DIP

This is a unanimously favorite recipe that always makes it to special gatherings because it is so good and easy to make. Baked tortilla chips, vegetables, and grains complement this versatile dip. Natural fresh salsas are available ready-made, or make your own for this recipe. Fantastic Foods makes the instant black bean or pinto bean mixes that I use for this dish. These convenient mixes are generally available in bulk at natural foods stores and they keep well.

INGREDIENTS	AMOUNT
butter (organic) or olive oil	2$\frac{1}{2}$ tsp.
cumin powder	1$\frac{1}{4}$ tsp.
turmeric powder	1$\frac{1}{4}$ tsp.
instant bean mix	1$\frac{1}{2}$ C.
pure water (boiling)	2 C.
fresh mild or hot salsa	2 C.
baked tortilla chips	
fresh and roasted vegetables	
fresh green herbs and feta cheese	

In a heavy iron skillet (8 inch), gently warm the butter or oil and stir in the cumin and turmeric. Turn off heat and stir in the instant bean mix. Add the boiling water, stir and cover tightly. Let stand for 15 to 20 minutes until thick. Stir and let cool. Combine the bean mix with the salsa. Serve in a large bowl in the center of a platter, and surround with baked tortilla chips, fresh vegetables, and cheese. Roasted vegetables can be combined with fresh vegetables for a grand effect! Makes 5 to 6 cups.

❀ BIG SCENE SALSA SALAD

Salsa and Bean Dip is great with grains too! Add the salsa to the bean mixture while it is still warm. Cook a seasonal grain such as rice, quinoa, millet, or barley. Combine $\frac{1}{2}$ cup dip with each 1$\frac{1}{2}$ cup cooked grain. Mound on

INGREDIENTS	AMOUNT
Salsa and Bean Dip (above)	$\frac{1}{2}$ C.
rice, quinoa, millet, or barley	1$\frac{1}{2}$ C.
pure water	3 C.
fresh greens	8 C.

a bed of fresh greens tossed with dressing. Garnish and serve. Very good! Serves 4.

✿ RUTABAGA AND SWEET POTATO SOUP

The flavor of this soup is very unique and comforting. The combination of rutabaga with potatoes is very healing for the stomach. I like to add the carrots, celery, parsley, and apples last, so the soup has a lightly cooked freshness. This way the live enzymes in foods, important for digestion, are left intact and the "life" is not cooked out of the soup.

INGREDIENTS	AMOUNT
onion (diced)	1 C.
mushrooms (sliced)	1 C.
water or broth	2½ C.
sweet potatoes (medium, quartered)	2
white potatoes (medium, quartered)	2
rutabaga (diced)	1½ C.
bay leaves	3
fresh rosemary	2 tsp. (1 tsp. dry)
cumin seeds	1½ tsp.
fresh turmeric	1 T. (1 tsp. dry)
fresh parsley (chopped)	¾ C.
carrots (medium, sliced)	2
celery (diced)	¾ C.
apple (small, diced)	1
fresh apple juice	2 C.
fresh garlic, tamari, flavored oil	garnish

In a stainless-steel soup pot, simmer the onion and mushrooms with ¼ cup water or broth until softened and lightly browned (15–20 minutes). Add the remaining water or broth, potatoes (do not peel), rutabaga, bay leaves, rosemary, cumin, and turmeric. Bring to a boil, cover and simmer until potatoes are soft, then add the parsley, carrots, and celery. Simmer for 5 more minutes and turn off the heat. Add the apple and apple juice, cover tightly and let stand for 20 minutes to meld the flavors. Garnish each bowl with a bit of fresh garlic and tamari or flavored oil, if desired. Serves 5.

✿ MOM'S CABBAGE SOUP WITH MILLET

My wonderful mother has always infused her cooking with love and caring, which produces very delicious results. When positive energy flows through the cook, it is transferred to the food and on to all who partake of it.

Mom's Cabbage Soup stands on its own, though I have added a favorite grain called millet. Millet is a treasure rarely found in the Western diet, a naturally "alkaline grain" higher in lysine (a building block for the immune system) than rice, corn, or oats. Millet will grow in harsh conditions with little water. Organic millet in bulk is found at natural foods stores. The trick to improving the flavor of millet is toasting the grain before cooking it.

INGREDIENTS	AMOUNT
yellow onion (diced)	$5^{1}/_{2}$ C.
cabbage (shredded)	8 C.
water or broth	2 quarts
oregano and marjoram	$2^{1}/_{2}$ tsp. each
tomato paste	3 T.
fresh tomatoes (crushed)	4 C.
red pepper (powder)	$^{1}/_{4}$ tsp.
molasses or maple syrup	$2^{1}/_{2}$ tsp.
millet (toasted)	1 C.
celery (diced)	2 C.
fresh basil leaves (minced)	$^{1}/_{3}$ C.
toasted sesame oil or olive oil	2 T.
tamari	to taste
garlic cloves (organic) (minced)	3
green onions	garnish

In a large stainless-steel soup pot, simmer the onion and cabbage in $^{1}/_{2}$ cup water or broth until softened and lightly browned (10 minutes). Add the oregano and marjoram and stir. Add the tomato paste, half of the fresh tomatoes, red pepper, remaining water or broth, and molasses or maple syrup. Bring to boil, cover and simmer for 15 to 20 minutes. In the meantime, heat a dry cast-iron skillet and add the millet. Stir the grain several times until evenly toasted to a light brown color. Add the millet to the soup pot, bring to boil, cover and simmer for 25 minutes. Turn the heat off and add the celery, fresh basil, oil, tamari, garlic, and the remaining fresh tomatoes. Cover the pot and let stand for 20 minutes to meld the flavors. Garnish each bowl with fresh green onions and enjoy! Serves 8 to 10.

✿ SESAME MILLET BURGERS WITH ROSEMARY PAN GRAVY

Millet is in my opinion the unsung hero of grains. It is a good source of protein, calcium, lecithin, iron, and B complex vitamins—not to mention its alkaline effect on the body. It is, however, not usually considered a winning choice for a dinner party. When this dish earned the coveted two-thumbs-up award at a special gathering, the recipe was adjusted to allow for second helpings! It can be prepared a day in advance during busy times. Take care to cover the mixture with a damp cloth and seal so that no air reaches it until you are ready to prepare the meal.

INGREDIENTS	AMOUNT
millet	2 C.
pure water	4 C.
carrots	4
garlic cloves (organic) (crushed)	3
sesame tahini	$1/4$ C.
egg (whole)	1
cumin powder	2 tsp.
paprika	2 tsp.
tamari	$1/4$ C.
Worcestershire sauce or prepared horseradish	$2^1/_2$ tsp.
tomatoes (diced)	$1/2$ C.
celery stalks (diced)	3
yellow onion (diced)	$1^1/_2$ C.
fresh basil or mixed fresh herbs	$1/3$ C.
toasted sesame oil (per burger)	1 tsp.
white sesame seeds (per burger)	1 tsp.
Rosemary Pan Gravy (p. 102)	

In a dry iron skillet, slowly toast the millet, stirring until lightly browned. Combine the millet and water in a saucepan, bring to boil, cover and simmer until tender (20 minutes). While the millet is cooking, slice the carrots into $1/8$-inch rounds and steam them in 1 cup water until tender (5 minutes). Save the carrot water for the gravy. In a blender jar, combine $3/4$ cup of the steamed carrots with the garlic, sesame tahini, egg, cumin, paprika, tamari, and Worcestershire sauce. Process until creamy. When the millet is done, let it cool. In a large bowl, mix the diced vegetables and herbs together so the flavors meld. When the millet is cooled, combine all ingredients together, including the remaining steamed carrots. The mixture should have the consistency of piecrust dough. Form firm, smooth patties (1 cup each) and place the millet burgers on parchment-lined cookie sheets. Smooth a teaspoon of toasted sesame oil on the top of each burger and sprinkle with sesame seeds. Bake at 325 degrees for 15 minutes, turn the heat down to 250 degrees and bake for another 20 minutes or until firm and lightly browned on top. Remove the burgers from the cookie sheet with a thin metal spatula. Serve the millet burgers topped with Rosemary Pan Gravy and a large salad of fresh greens. Serves 5 to 7.

✿ ROSEMARY PAN GRAVY

A rich-tasting broth is essential for making a variety of good gravies, sauces, and soups. Natural foods stores usually stock good-quality powdered broth bases that are quick and easy to use. I use onion powder to enrich the broth base for this recipe, and always prefer the highly nutritious kuzu root starch over other thickening agents.

INGREDIENTS	AMOUNT
garlic cloves or shallots	2
rich broth base	2¹/₂ C.
fresh rosemary leaves (minced)	2 T.
kuzu root powder	1 T.
cold water	2 T.
tamari	1 T.
paprika	2 tsp.

Mince the garlic or shallots and brown lightly in a pan sprinkled with 2 or 3 tablespoons broth or water. Add the carrot water (from steamed carrots) and enough broth or plain water to make 2¹/₂ cups liquid. If using plain water, enrich it with broth powder until the taste reaches the desired intensity. Add the fresh rosemary and simmer for 5 minutes. Make a thin paste in a small bowl by combining the kuzu with the cold water. Bring the gravy to a boil and stir in the starch paste until gravy is thickened. Remove from heat and stir in the tamari and paprika. Rosemary Pan Gravy is great over steamed vegetables and grains, baked potatoes, or squash, and of course Sesame Millet Burgers!

✿ EGGPLANT WITH CHILI TAMARI SAUCE

Eggplant, native to Thailand and Eastern India, is perhaps the most elegant member of the tomato family. It comes in different sizes, shapes, and colors and is a good substitute for meat in many dishes. Eggplant can be grilled for a smoky flavor, baked, simmered, or stir-fried. The versatile nature of this member of the nightshade family makes it ideal for combining with garlic, basil, curry, and chilies. Eggplant should be well-cooked or it will have a bitter flavor.

Rinse the rice and dry roast it in a heavy iron skillet (no oil) until lightly browned. Add the water and simmer until rice is tender (about 40 minutes). While the rice is cooking, wash the skin of the eggplants with soap and rinse. Cut the tops off, then slice into even strips about ¹/₄-inch thick and 3 inches long. Soak the eggplant strips in cold water for 15 minutes and drain. Put the eggplant in a stainless-steel sauté pan or wok. Add ¹/₄ cup onion broth or stock, cover and simmer until eggplant is tender (about 30 minutes). Add the basil and green onion or chives, leaving enough aside for a garnish. Cover, and remove from heat. Make the sauce in a small pan using the remaining onion broth, tamari, and thai chili paste. Mix the kuzu root powder with enough cold water to thin it. Bring the sauce to a boil and stir in the starch until sauce is thickened; add the olive oil and maple syrup. Stir the sauce into the eggplant and serve over the rice. Garnish the top with the remaining basil and onion. This dish is very good with a cabbage salad, or use two red chard leaves per plate. Arrange the rice and eggplant on top of the chard, leaving a colorful border. Serves 6.

INGREDIENTS	AMOUNT
brown rice or jasmine rice	2 C.
pure water	4 C.
purple globe eggplant (medium)	2
onion powder broth or stock	$3/4$ C.
fresh basil (chopped)	1 C.
green onion or chives	$1/2$ C.
tamari	$1/3$ C.
thai chili paste or chili flakes	2 tsp.
kuzu root, arrowroot, or cornstarch	2 to 3 tsp.
roasted garlic olive oil	$1/4$ C.
maple syrup	$1^1/2$ tsp.
red chard leaves (optional)	12

✺ ECLIPSE OF THE MOON BROWN BETTY

This is a great dish to make when the oven is needed to bake a casserole or potatoes in the colder months. The rich, nutlike flavor of this unique pie will delight the senses any time; it is especially good served warm. With a crown of whipped cream flavored with vanilla and rum, this could take the place of a birthday cake, and it is good for you too! This recipe was created during the night of a full eclipse of the moon.

Use canola or grapeseed oil to lightly coat the bottom and sides of a 9-inch glass baking casserole (with cover). Wash, core, and dice (do not peel) the apples and pears. Put them

INGREDIENTS	AMOUNT
canola or grapeseed oil	1 tsp.
Granny Smith apples	3 C.
bosc pears	3 C.
rolled oats, divided	1 C.
maple syrup	$1/4$ C.
brown rice syrup	$1/3$ C.
pure water	$1/4$ C.
lemon juice	1 T.
lemon rind	2 tsp.
nutmeg and cinnamon	2 tsp. each
powdered cloves	$1/8$ tsp.
flaxseed	$1/3$ C.
shelled walnuts	$1/2$ C.

into the baking dish and toss with $^1/_3$ cup of the rolled oats. In a separate bowl, combine the syrups, water, lemon juice and rind, and spices, then stir half of this mixture into the fruit. Put the flaxseed, walnuts, and $^1/_2$ cup of the rolled oats in a nut grinder or blender and process to a flour. Combine the flour with the remaining syrup mixture. Crumble this evenly over the fruit and sprinkle the remaining oats over the top. Cover and bake at 325 degrees for about 35 minutes, then uncover and bake for 10 more minutes or until tender and brown. Serves 6.

FROZEN BANANA ICE CREAMS

There is growing evidence that a diet rich in potassium eases hypertension, or high blood pressure. Bananas and other fruits such as cantaloupe, honeydew, oranges, and grapefruit are high in both fiber and potassium. Frozen banana ice creams are a wonderful alternative to commercially prepared ice cream products. The variations are endless and best of all they take only minutes to prepare if you have a blender. Frozen banana ice creams always get rave reviews! Simply peel ripe bananas, and keep them in the freezer where they remain ready for these quick, healthy desserts.The following dessert recipes are elegant enough to serve at a special dinner party, and simple enough for a snack.

✿ BANANA COCONUT ICE CREAM

Slice frozen bananas into coins and place in blender with remaining ingredients. Process until creamy. Serve in martini glasses. Garnish with toasted coconut or a sprinkle of nutmeg. Serves 3 to 4.

INGREDIENTS	AMOUNT
frozen bananas	3
lowfat coconut milk	$^1/_3$ C.
heavy cream or apple juice	2 T.
nutmeg	$^1/_4$ tsp.
raspberry jam (sugarless)	1 T.
toasted coconut	garnish

✿ BANANA WALNUT ICE CREAM

Put walnuts, cream or juice, and vanilla in blender and process; then add frozen bananas cut into coins. Garnish with extra walnuts and sauce of choice. Serves 4.

INGREDIENTS	AMOUNT
fresh-shelled walnuts	$^1/_4$ C.
cream or apple juice	$^1/_3$ C.
vanilla	1 tsp.
frozen bananas	3

CHAPTER FIVE

AUTUMN RESTORATION

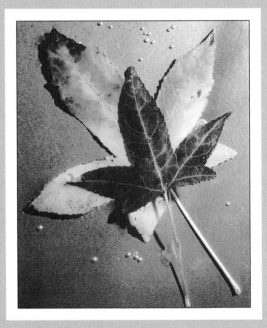

CONSCIOUSNESS CREATES REALITY
INDIVIDUALLY, AND COLLECTIVELY.[1]

—CAZEKIEL

INTROSPECTIVE AUTUMN

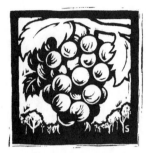

Autumn is a most important time for major cleansing. Like early spring, early autumn is a key time for cleansing, but in this season your diet may be fuller, richer, and more heat-producing than in spring—in order to carry you through the chill of late autumn and winter.

Metal is associated with autumn. It represents the mineral ores and salts of Earth. The **lungs** and the **large intestine** are the two body organs associated with the Metal element, and the tissues of the body governed by Metal are the skin and body hair. Thus, Metal fortifies the skin and hair, and their health often reflects that of the lungs and large intestine. In fact, the skin acts as the third lung, absorbing from the environment and expiring wastes into the air. In both Chinese and Western medicines, lung and skin problems are seen as closely related. The lungs and the large intestine are the organs stimulated to cleanse in autumn. So, to help strengthen the body and deflect winter illness, a fast for the large intestine is indispensable.

THE LUNGS

Breathing involves both the intake of new air (energy) during inhalation and the elimination of the old air (waste) in exhalation. The Buddhists see each in-breath giving new life and each out-breath as a little death. Thus, your deepest attitudes toward living and dying may affect your breathing process and the health of the Metal element in your body.

Our lungs communicate between the inner and outer atmospheres. Asthma, eczema, and skin rashes are commonly associated with colds and lung infections, and dry or oily skin may also suggest an imbalance. Just as proper food is needed for energy and health, deep breathing and clean air are vital to life.

With every breath we take, etheric energy is also taken in. This etheric energy is what the yogis call *prana*, which means "etheric." Prana has two polarities—positive and negative—and our bodies make use of both energies. Through the right nostril we inhale positive prana, through the left nostril we inhale negative prana. Both are needed for our well-being.

The right or positive current of prana is called the solar energy, and the left or negative current is called the lunar energy. The positive solar energy being drawn through the right nostril can be used for self-vitalization by placing a piece of cotton in your left nostril and breathing only through the right one for about one hour. During this time, center your thoughts upon the part of your body that needs rebuilding or rejuvenating. This breathing technique, coupled with focused thought, is very powerful—you will be surprised at what happens.

It is known that great natural healers breathe for greater periods of time through the right nostril; they are able to extract and utilize more solar energy this way and therefore do not exhaust themselves as readily.

It is a good practice to make a habit of breathing through the right nostril when we eat. The solar current, the positive prana, speeds up the process of metabolism. Then we can extract most of the energy from the food we eat, so we eat less and are satisfied. On the other hand, when undergoing a fast, block the right nostril and breathe more through the left. You will not become as hungry because your metabolism will slow down. In the East, all yogis practice this technique when they go on long fasts. The various techniques of breathing, discussed in studies of yoga, can be very time-consuming. However, if we remember that when we inhale we take in the pranic energies, then we can train ourselves to inhale slowly and deeply.

SIMPLE BREATHING EXERCISE

1. Inhale and hold your breath to the count of 4, then exhale.
2. Repeat for 10 breaths or more, increasing the number of breaths slowly.

Certain breaths are used for stimulating the various functions of the body. Science declares that everything we require for the building of our body tissue is held in suspension in the air. It is calculated that without the influence of prana, of magnetic and other forces, we could not live. We could eat day and night, yet starve to death because we could not extract enough energies from the food and drink we consume.

When we inhale and fill our lungs with air, the etheric energy is extracted and is drawn into the fourth-dimensional tubes that lie to the right and left sides of the spine. The right tube is called *Pingala;* it starts at the right nostril and extends down the right side of the spine. *Ida* starts at the left nostril and extends down the left side of the spine. Pingala, the right tube, draws the positive current while Ida, the left tube, draws the negative current. We draw these currents alternately: One hour we draw positive current and the next hour we draw negative current. When we become disturbed emotionally, we throw this system out of balance and neglect to draw the energies in the proper proportions.

When we think of the power of breath and how essential it is to our well-being, we should place more importance on the study and practice of taking in life currents, energies, and supplies for the body. It is an inexpensive way to attain the building blocks for our bodies. Conscious breathing should be taught and practiced in every household. The demand for fresh, lead-free, and unpolluted air is highly justified; in polluted—lead-, nicotine-, and chemical-laden air—the vital current of prana is reduced to 2 percent. In general, this makes us easily exhausted and tired; besides not getting enough oxygen, we cannot extract enough prana from the air. Only through this divinely intelligent arrangement of the positive and negative can the body live and have its being.

PINEAPPLE FAST FOR THE LUNGS

A good fast to help heal the lungs is located on page 129.

GARLIC

An important herb for cleansing and feeding the lungs is garlic, an herb deeply rooted in our folk medicine and one that has been used for centuries. Early pyramid builders ate garlic daily for endurance, while the Greeks used it to cure snakebite and pneumonia. During World War I, garlic was used extensively to prevent gangrene and to treat typhus and dysentery. Certain Slavic peoples still eat a clove of raw garlic with each meal during the winter months to prevent colds and flu.

In 1858 Louis Pasteur confirmed that garlic juice killed bacteria in laboratory culture dishes, and modern research has confirmed garlic's ability to bolster the human immune system. Japanese researchers have shown that garlic can prevent infection by the influenza virus. Several studies have also shown that garlic destroys the virus that causes cold sores. A 1984 study at Georgetown University Hospital found that whole garlic extract halted the growth of 30 strains of bacteria, including 6 strains that cause tuberculosis.

It is well known today that garlic is an effective treatment for internal and external infections; it acts by combining with harmful bacteria to stop their action, allowing healthful bacteria to proliferate. It is a specific for bronchitis, asthma, high blood pressure, stomach ulcers, chronic colitis, influenza, urinary tract infections, *Candida albicans*, cardiovascular problems, and all respiratory infections including colds. As a preventive, it has no equal in the home.

At the faintest sign of sore throat, running nose, or aching bones, simply peel a clove of fresh garlic, cut it in half, and place one half in each cheek, allowing the juice to be absorbed in the saliva and pervade the system. The odor can be masked by use of anise, cinnamon, or caraway seeds; chew these with a little parsley. Both garlic tablets and capsules are available for those who cannot adjust to the garlic odor, but fresh garlic is always preferred for the live enzymes it contains. Commercially grown garlic may be treated with a variety of chemical sprays. Therefore, organically grown garlic is preferred.

The following methods of preparing garlic for home use are easy and effective recipes excerpted from the book *Herbs, Partners in Life* by Adelle G. Dawson.[2]

❧ OIL OF GARLIC

Peel and mince 1 cup of garlic. Put in a jar and cover with warm olive oil. Turn the jar several times a day for 4 days; then strain the oil. Store the garlic oil in a cool place; use the minced garlic for garlic bread and in salads or steamed vegetables. The oil can be taken in 1 teaspoon doses 3 or 4 times daily, or used in dressings for salads and vegetable dishes.

❧ GARLIC COUGH MEDICINE

Place 1 pound of peeled and sliced garlic in a jar, and cover with a mixture of equal parts apple cider vinegar and water. Let stand for 4 or 5 hours, strain, and add an equal amount of honey. Keep in a cool place and shake well before using. One tablespoon may be taken 3 or 4 times a day.

For bronchitis, put 2 whole, peeled cloves of garlic through a press; add to 1 cup of maple syrup or honey; take the entire cupful, a spoonful at a time, during a 24-hour period.

❧ GARLIC BANDAGE

Fresh grated garlic or expressed juice may be put directly on any external wound or infection. In World War I, the army discovered the efficacy of garlic as a disinfectant for wounds, and it was credited with saving many lives.

❧ GARLIC VINEGAR

The famous "Four Thieves Vinegar" is an example of the immunity to disease that garlic gives. During the plague of 1722, four thieves in the city of Marseilles achieved immunity through daily doses of garlic vinegar, which allowed them to plunder the dead bodies of plague victims without contracting the disease. Garlic vinegar is made by leaving sliced cloves of garlic to marinate in apple cider vinegar.

GARLIC WISDOM

No household should ever be without a good supply of fresh garlic. If you have even a small garden, garlic is easy to grow and harvest. Divide the bulb into its separate cloves and plant in the fall in well-tilled, rich, well-drained loamy soil. The garlic will be ready to harvest the following July when the tops begin to turn yellow. Cure the bulbs for 2 to 4 weeks in a dark, dry area where the temperature is moderate.

In using garlic in a healthy diet, remember that boiling destroys medicinal properties. Add it to soups, stews, vegetables, and salads just before serving. Always use garlic or ginger with meats to counter the toxic acids meats create during digestion. Garlic bread has long been considered a gourmet addition to a crisp green salad or homemade soup.

Other herbs used for respiratory ailments include angelica, black mustard, burdock, coltsfoot, comfrey, eucalyptus, fenugreek, hyssop, licorice, lobelia, mullein, pine, sunflower, thyme, walnut, witch hazel, and yerba santa.

THE SKIN

The thyroid gland located at the base of the neck controls all functions of the body's three layers of skin: the outer skin called the hide; the inner skin called the mucous membrane; and a middle skin, the serous membrane, which lines the pleural, pericardial, peritoneal, and cranial cavities and also the joints.

The normal functions of the outer skin are to exhale gases, sweat out water and certain toxic salty substances, oil the skin and its hair with special oil glands, and protect the inner body. The elimination, which results from forcefully exuding gases, acid sweat, and toxic oils and gases through the outer skin, has supplied names to enough diseases to fill a large dermatology textbook. Chronic eczema, ichthyosis, and psoriasis are common examples. Skin diseases, which are really signs of toxic irritation, respond well to treatment—dietary and local—directed toward neutralization and elimination of the offending poisons.

The inner skin, or mucous membrane, normally secretes a clear mucus that keeps the membranes moist and, with the aid of the flagellated lining cells, propels irritants and foreign bodies toward an elimination point. Under duress, the thyroid gland may force toxins out through the mucous cells.

When only the superficial cells of the inner skin are involved and the secretion is watery, the illness is called a cold or catarrh. As the deeper layers are affected, the discharge becomes muco-purulent (mucus and pus), purulent (pure pus), or purulent-hemorrhagic (pus and blood). Under these headings would come such illnesses as sinusitis, bronchitis, gastritis, enteritis, appendicitis, tonsillitis, mastitis, cervicitis, pyelitis, and any other "itis" where inflammation of the mucous or serous membrane occurs.

Researchers are discovering that a variety of skin problems indicate major or minor nutritional deficiencies. To identify underlying nutritional problems before they get started, watch your skin for warning signs to help pinpoint dietary needs.

Here are some common deficiencies and how they show up on your skin.

1. Vitamin C shortage—bleeding gums, soreness in mouth and gums, or a rough, scaly rash around hair roots.
2. Vitamin B complex deficiency—cracks and canker sores in the corners of the mouth.
3. Dry skin and brittle nails are often due to a lack of cold-pressed oils and essential fatty-acid oils such as omega-3 and omega-6 in the diet.

FASTING ON GRAPES

TIME: Fall
TIME FRAME: 3 to 4 days

Grapes contain an extraordinary class of bioflavonoids called proanthocyanidins, which are many times more powerful than vitamins C and E at scavenging free radicals. They are also packed with antioxidant phytochemicals (health-enhancing chemicals in plants), which promote cellular health by neutralizing carcinogens and boosting the activity of detoxifying enzymes.

The exceptional properties of the grape also promote blood vessel health by protecting the strength and flexibility of collagen structures—the fibrous proteins in blood vessels, tissue cells, gums, bones, and teeth. Furthermore, grapes help protect the collagen structures that give skin its smoothness and elasticity. They are naturally high in the mineral silicon, which is also a part of the connective tissue of skin, hair, and nails.

The grape is Nature's most complex fruit. We find that grapes, both as a mono-diet and in packs (see below), have figured in restorative health therapies in Europe for more than 6,000 years. They seem to be particularly helpful in treating tumors and some cancers. Colored grapes such as concord are preferable to the green variety. They are eaten or juiced in large quantities over a 3- to 4-day period, withholding any other food or drink. This can be done each month if needed. Utilize the internal bath of your choice to clear the system while fasting on grapes.

Simple grape packs are made by lightly crushing grapes and packing them $1/2$ to $1^1/2$ inches thick between layers of cloth or directly on the skin. Apply to the external areas of affected inner organs and tissues for 1 to 4 hours each day, for ulcers in the stomach and duodenum as well as inflammatory conditions in the cecum and appendix areas. Naturopathic institutes apply grape poultices on cancerous areas of the body.

HERBS FOR SKIN CANCER AND SUNBURN

Herbs used for skin cancer can be taken internally as teas or capsules, and can also be applied externally as compresses and plasters. These herbs include bitterroot, cabbage, chaparral, dandelion, echinacea, garlic, goldenseal, lobelia, mandrake, mullein, red clover, sage, slippery elm, sorrel, tansy, and walnut.

Herbs for treating sunburn include aloe vera, aspen, beech, birch, cattail, comfrey, echinacea, elderberry, horsetail, juniper, red clover, slippery elm, and yarrow. Dr. Christopher's Beauty Facial Cream is the best herbal cream I know of to care for your skin (see Sources).

❧ CABBAGE SOUP FAST FOR BEAUTY
TIME: Fall and Winter
TIME FRAME: 1 to 3 days

This drink is rich in iron, calcium, magnesium, and phosphorus. The flaxseed or hempseed oil is optional but should be included if you have dry skin or brittle nails. Cabbage

INGREDIENTS	AMOUNT
fresh cabbage	1 small
pure water	1½ to 2 C.
lemon (organic)	1
flaxseed or hempseed oil	optional

water is a folk remedy and is very good for bad skin.

Wash cabbage, cut in half. Put half of the cabbage head in a saucepan with the water, cover and simmer for 20 minutes, cool and strain. Pour the cabbage water into a wide-mouth jar, and eat the warm cabbage. One hour after eating the cabbage, put the other half of the cabbage through a juicer with the lemon (include rind). Add the fresh cabbage juice to the boiled cabbage water; drink ½ cup every other hour until it is finished. Herbal teas, such as sage and red clover, go well with this fast, as does barley water.

❧ BARLEY WATER
Barley water is pleasant to drink, soothing for the stomach, and excellent for dry blotchy skin when taken regularly.

Wash barley, place in saucepan with the water, cover and simmer. After barley has simmered for 30

INGREDIENTS	AMOUNT
pearl barley (organic)	½ C.
pure water	3½ C.
fresh lemon peel (organic only)	½
honey or maple syrup	if desired

minutes, add the fresh lemon peel and continue cooking for an additional 30 minutes. Strain the liquid from the barley while still hot; cool before bottling and store in refrigerator. Take ½ cup 3 times a day with 1 teaspoon of sweetener if desired. Reserve cooked barley, add to soups and stews. Makes 3 cups.

🌿 SAGE TEA

Sage flowers attract bees, which produce wonderful sage honey. The tea is an excellent beauty beverage, pleasant to drink, and a blood purifier.

Bring water to a boil, remove from heat and add sage leaves. Cover tightly and steep 6 to 8 minutes;

INGREDIENTS	AMOUNT
pure water	2 C.
dried sage leaves	2 or 3 T.
(double if fresh)	
orange juice	to taste

strain and add a few drops of orange juice for flavor. Take ½ cup 3 times a day before or after meals.

THE LARGE INTESTINE

The large intestine, also known as the colon or bowel, is one organ that is generally not considered or discussed when problems arise regarding the health of an individual. But, in today's society, it is often congested through our selection of inadequate foods and improper preparation methods. Recent research reveals that various strains of virus, bacteria, and parasites establish themselves in the cecum—a saclike organ connecting the small and large intestines. These undesirable—and often undetected—guests can cause recurring illness and wreak havoc in the system.

Congestion of the large intestine, both acute and chronic, often leads to the organ's prolapse and loss of tone and is the cause of many pains and illnesses. General abdominal discomfort and low- and mid-backaches are often referred pain from the distention of the large intestine. Pressure in the head and sinuses, headaches, sore throats, crankiness, lack of energy, and even lack of enthusiasm for life, can result from congestion in this organ.

Lack of fiber in the diet increases the transit time of wastes through the colon and allows production of putrefactive bacteria. Both of these factors have been linked to diseases such as colitis, diverticulosis, cancer, and other chronic diseases of the body. The *Merck Manual,* the medical industry's standard text for the diagnosis and treatment of disease, states that colon degeneration is on the rise. The incidence of diverticulosis (bowel pockets) has increased dramatically over the past 50 years. In 1993 almost half of U.S. adults were found to have herniation of the large intestine.

A general assumption is that the large intestine will take care of itself. In times past, knowledge of how to care for the large intestine was more widespread and accepted. Knowing how to keep this important organ healthy and in good shape allows us to guard ourselves from disease and illness.

Health specialists say that there is only one disease—*constipation*. Not just constipation of the colon, but clogging of all internal organs. The colon is one of our chief waste disposal plants. When the colon is clean and working properly, the rest of the body, including all our organs, is free to clean house and dump into the waste stream, so to speak. If the colon is clogged with waste, other glands and organs become bogged down with toxins and unwanted mucus; some of them cease or nearly cease functioning. In many cases, the result is removal of the gland or organ by surgery.

Note: Refer to the internal bath section (chapter 7) for a more detailed perspective regarding the colon, and particularly before beginning your fast for the large intestine. The cleansing diet for the large intestine is one of the most useful and important fasts to improve overall health. Once the system is relieved of the burdensome toxic waste, the body can assimilate nutrients more readily, and it becomes more responsive to other cleansing fasts as well as the good foods you eat.

COLON CARE ESSENTIALS

An article in *Science News* suggests that the cecum area in the colon is a site that may be a contributing factor to persistent infections and to progressive infections. Bacteria establish colonies in the cecum, a large sack or structure at the junction of the small and large intestines (vol. 150, Oct. 5, 1996).

Signs of colon congestion can be sinus and lung build-up with excess mucus, respiratory problems, allergies, earache, sore throat, bronchitis, strong body odor (including feet), and constipation. Before you begin this amazing cleansing fast, it would be useful to read the following descriptions for the large intestine and note which best describe the state of your intestinal health. Once you determine your condition, it is possible to achieve the best results while fasting for the large intestine.

ATONIC COLON: *Atonic* means "lack of tone." The colon is loose, flaccid, and sluggish; it balloons and stretches, but will move on a regular basis. Transit time is slow.

NEEDS: raw foods, coarse fibers, apples, calcium for tone; stimulant (bitter) laxatives—cascara sagrada, senna; also barberry, buckthorn bark, black walnut hulls, bran, psyllium hulls, alfalfa, marsh mallow, and pepsin.

SPASTIC COLON: Tends to move very irregularly, sporadic (muscle spasms). Instead of cascara sagrada or senna, use gentle laxatives such as licorice root with catnip, castor oil, or Epsom salts. Instead of psyllium hulls, use psyllium seed, flaxseed, slippery elm, fruit pectin, and oat bran. Good herbal teas include comfrey, Irish moss, mullein, marsh mallow, and buckthorn bark.

NEEDS: lightly steamed vegetables, gentle fiber foods such as raw wheat germ, rice, millet, nuts, seeds, and fruits. Too much calcium can constipate; use magnesium to relax muscles, and B vitamins and relaxing herbal teas such as the mints, lobelia, scullcap, and Oregon grape root.

COMBINATION: Some individuals may experience a combination of atonic and spastic colon. In this case, use a combination of the foods listed until comfortable results are achieved.

COMMON: Other common abnormalities of the colon include adhesions, ballooning, colitis, diverticulosis (bowel pockets), prolapsus, ulceration, and mucosal dysfunction. If you suspect that you have any of these conditions, consult your health practitioner before undergoing pressurized colonic treatment. In conditions such as adhesions and ulceration, the aloe vera and flaxseed healing waters are very soothing. Prolapsus is helped by the daily use of the slant board in connection with massage. (The slant board is available by mail order through Living Arts. See Sources. Or you can make your own using a padded board to support your body.) Elevate one end 12 to 18 inches. Lie on the board with your feet elevated. This reverses the gravity and increases blood flow to the brain. Allow your body to guide you as to how much time you should lie with your feet elevated higher than your head. Sleeping on the slant board is beneficial for most healthy individuals. (Dr. Bernard Jensen is a good source for more extensive information on this subject. See Sources.) If diverticulitis is present, use the Cascara Sagrada Tea (p. 180), along with massage, in place of colon or enema therapies. Herbs for bowel pockets include barberry, black haw, black walnut, cascara sagrada, fennel, garlic, gingerroot, goldenseal, lobelia, and wormwood.

❧ CLEANSING FAST FOR THE LARGE INTESTINE

I call this fast for the large intestine *Plumbarius* (Latin for "plumber") because the cleansing action on the body may be likened to the results that a plumber gets when opening up a clogged drain. Everything moves better. My first encounter with fasting involved an elaborate 6-day fast directed to the large intestine; it appeared to yield only minor results. I was disappointed, but after becoming ill about six weeks later, I did try the colon cleansing fast again. About the third day, I was stunned when the old, rubbery, and foul waste was expelled with the assistance of the internal baths (chapter 7). The results were amazing. With the help of improved diet, allergies disappeared, energy returned, skin improved, night sweats disappeared, yearly colds became much less severe and less frequent. Best of all, I experienced a calm and clear sensation of peace and well-being. So, if at first you do not succeed, try again! Your good efforts will be rewarded sevenfold.

This is a detailed version of this special cleanse, but it is actually very simple. If you prefer a less extensive cleanse, go to the Simple Colon Cleanse on page 122.

This cleanse helps the body become more receptive to all other fasts by relieving it of toxic mucus accumulation. Once successfully completed, there is no need to do this fast each year if you maintain a proper diet. After completion of the fast, your elimination pattern may change, but it will return to normal when a new mucous lining forms. Foods high in fiber, such as whole grains, are vital to tone the newly cleansed colon. Take a moment to familiarize yourself with the basic ingredients needed to gain a clear understanding of the process.

TIME: Autumn
TIME FRAME: 3 to 5 days

WHAT YOU WILL NEED AND WHY
1. Epsom salts to empty the digestive tract and an enema bag to finish the job. Your local drugstore is a good source for these. If they do not carry enema bags, ask to have one ordered.
2. 6 oranges, 2 limes, 6 grapefruit, 2 lemons (these are used 1 day only with the Epsom salts to cleanse the digestive tract and hydrate the body).
3. A natural bristle skin brush with a long handle to reach your back.
4. Niacin tablets (50 mgs) to promote increased blood and lymphatic circulation.
5. Herbs for teas, such as red clover, blessed thistle, and yellow dock root. These herbs used in combination help improve nutrient absorption and assist the body's natural cleansing process. Herbs to help balance the system and provide strength and nou-

INGREDIENTS	AMOUNT
red clover, hawthorn leaf and flowers,	3 T.
alfalfa leaf, nettles, sage, horsetail,	
echinacea, milk thistle seed, pau d'arco,	
gotu kola, lemongrass, blue malva, and	
yerba santa.	
pure water	2 C.

rishment during a cleanse are used in this delightful combination known as Cleansing and Fasting Tea. It is available from Crystal Star Herbal Nutrition (see Sources). Or it can be mixed dry and stored until needed.

Use equal parts of the herbs listed. Follow the basic method of steeping 3 tablespoons of herbs in 2 cups of pure water that has been boiled; allow from 10 to 30 minutes for the tea to steep, tightly covered so that the volatile oils will not escape.

Drink teas throughout the day rather than all at once to allow more absorption of the nutrients. When correctly used, herbs promote the elimination of waste matter and toxins from the body by simple, natural means. They are easily absorbed by the body as liquid, which provides gentle flushing action, releasing herbal energy that supports Nature in its fight against disease. Herbal teas are the most basic and ancient of all therapeutic mediums.

6. Fresh live apple juice from apples that are organically grown and fresh-pressed. Avoid the clear type or canned. You will need 1 to 2 quarts depending on the length of your fast. The apple juice is diluted with water, so 1 quart is stretched to 2 quarts. The natural pectin in apple juice helps soften and loosen hardened matter in the digestive tract and is excellent for its cleansing effects and compatibility with intestinal brooming aids (see below).

7. Intestinal brooming aids are natural fibers used in cleansing; psyllium seed hulls are one of the most effective. The tiny seeds of the psyllium flower so resemble a flea that the plant's name was derived from the ancient Greek word for flea. One genus grows wild in southern Europe, North Africa, and Asia, where it is still known as "flea seed" because of its small, glossy, dark brown seeds. A hairy-stemmed variety, native to India and Iran, produces tiny blond seeds. The tiny husk of blond psyllium seed has a widespread reputation for helping to improve gastrointestinal ailments such as constipation, cystitis, diarrhea, and dysentery. Composed almost entirely of hemicellulose, psyllium husks have the highest bulking activity of any of the major dietary fibers. By binding with water in the intestines, psyllium increases the bulk and softness of intestinal contents; it absorbs toxins, soothes inflamed tissues, and promotes the growth of friendly colonic bacteria. This herb also helps to eliminate bile acids and lowers harmful blood cholesterol. Plain whole psyllium husks may be used, or there are pleasant alternatives such as combining them with slippery elm, chia, or flaxseed for those who find they do not handle psyllium husks well. The body needs a balance of

soluble and insoluble fibers. Each has a special set of functions to keep the body healthy, as in the following psyllium combination.

❧ PSYLLIUM-OAT-PECTIN POWDER

This is my recipe for a good-quality, inexpensive, and healthy intestinal broom powder for your autumn cleansing fast.

INGREDIENTS	AMOUNT
oat bran	$^1/_4$ C.
flaxseed	2 T.
psyllium hulls	1 C.
fruit pectin	1 T.

Place the oat bran and flaxseed in a blender or nut grinder and process to a powder.

Mix dry ingredients together and blend well. Store the powder in a glass container with a screw top and refrigerate. Use 1 heaping teaspoon at a time, as called for in the apple cleansing drinks you will have for your fast.

Note: If you have a spastic colon, or if psyllium is too strong in its action, and therefore constipating to your system, replace it with slippery elm bark powder or a combination of the psyllium and slippery elm bark powder in equal parts. Allergic reactions to psyllium are rare, but they can occur. If you develop a strange allergic reaction, such as a red rash or swelling, substitute the herb slippery elm. Be sure to check with your professional consultant immediately if you react negatively to psyllium.

8. Slippery elm is a nutritive herb indigenous to the Americas and was one of the herbs most used by Native Americans of the eastern seaboard and high plains areas. They used it as an important survival food. Slippery elm's gentle lubricating effect is beneficial to the whole body; it also absorbs cholesterol, carcinogenic compounds, heavy metals, and toxic materials. It strengthens, heals, and soothes inflamed or irritated areas, absorbs noxious gases, neutralizes stomach acidity, and soothes irritated sore throats, gastrointestinal ulcers, and dryness of the respiratory tract. It will usually stay down when all else causes nausea and vomiting.

   Slippery elm is equal to oatmeal in vitamin and mineral content—high in B complex vitamins and protein, with moderate amounts of vitamin A and selenium, and small amounts of vitamins E and K and the mineral magnesium. It contains trace amounts of iron, phosphorus, zinc, potassium, silicon, and sodium.

9. Liquid bentonite is a special clay of volcanic ash, hydrated and suspended in water by a scientific process, resulting in a product called Sonne's No. 7. This clay aids in the detoxification of the alimentary canal by absorbing many times its own weight in positive- and negative-charged ions. The product is carried by many natural foods stores.

10. Whey powder feeds the acidophilus and bifidus bacteria in the intestines and prevents the development of harmful putrefactive bacteria, which leads to autotoxemia. Whey contains rich amounts of B complex vitamins and serves as nutritional support during your fast.

Important Note: To achieve successful results with this cleansing fast, the use of enema therapy or colonic irrigation is essential. Chapter 7 explains these valuable internal bath therapies. No solid food is eaten during this fast. If you eat solid food, this fast will not work. Each day should begin with skin brushing for 3 to 5 minutes (refer to chapter 7).

DAY 1:
1. Skin brush in the morning. Plan to be near a rest room for the first day of your fast.
2. Dissolve 1 tablespoon of Epsom salts in $\frac{1}{4}$ cup warm water and $\frac{1}{4}$ cup citrus juice. Drink the Epsom salts water. This saline solution creates a laxative effect, which clears out the system and prepares it for the apple cleansing drinks.
3. To keep the body well-hydrated during this process, combine the juice of the 6 oranges and the 2 limes with enough water to make $1\frac{1}{2}$ quarts. Drink 1 or 2 cups, slowly, every $\frac{1}{2}$ hour until it is finished. Repeat, using the 6 grapefruit and the 2 lemons. The laxative effect from the salt will continue through the day with the aid of the juices.
4. When the citrus juices are finished, take an enema to clear out any remaining matter before bedtime (chapter 7).
5. Before going to sleep, take your first cleansing drink consisting of apple juice, bentonite, and psyllium (recipe below). Then drink a cup of herbal tea or juice. You should sleep well.

🍂 APPLE CLEANSING DRINK

This is the main cleansing drink you will have 5 times each day.

In a glass container, which serves well as a drinking cup and has a tight fitting lid, combine the ingredients. Put the lid on and shake the container to mix the ingredients well. There should be no

INGREDIENTS	AMOUNT
apple juice (organic)	$^1/_2$ C.
pure water	$^1/_3$ C.
bentonite	1 tsp.
whey powder	1 tsp.
psyllium or slippery elm powder	1 heaping tsp.
or intestinal cleanser of choice	
(atonic-spastic)	

lumps. Drink this mixture before it thickens too much. Then rinse the container out and set it to dry for your next drink, taken 3 hours later. Herbal teas, broths, and fresh juices can be enjoyed as desired between the 3-hour intervals, until a total of 5 apple-cleansing drinks per day has been taken (schedule example: 7 A.M. - 10 A.M. - 1 P.M. - 4 P.M. - 7 P.M.).

DAYS 2 THROUGH 6:

1. Skin brush in the morning. Plan to rest or do light work. (Apple cleansing drink ingredients can travel: combine the juice, bentonite, and water; keep the powder separate and add before drinking.)
2. Take the first of 5 apple-cleansing drinks first thing in the morning.
3. Between the 3-hour intervals, you can enjoy all of the herbal teas, broths, or fresh-pressed juices you desire; it is essential to take extra liquids with the apple cleansing drinks to ensure proper hydration for the brooming aids.
4. Take two niacin tablets beginning on the second day of the fast. Repeat two or three times daily during the fast, between apple cleansing drinks. You should feel a niacin "flush" where the body tingles and the skin reddens—a good time to take a steam bath to flush toxins out through the skin. If you do not feel the "flush," increase the dosage of niacin slightly. This step is optional and may be omitted if preferred. Baths are also optional, but are highly beneficial.
5. Internal baths are important in this fast. The apple cleansing drinks will soften the hardened matter, or intestinal plaque, in the colon and the impactions are loosened by stimulation of the enema or colonic. Usually by the third or fourth day of fasting, impacted matter that has been lining your colon for years will empty out in long (3 to 5 foot) ropes shaped like the colon, rubberlike (resembling a

wrinkled-up tube), and foul. This lining is made of layers of mucus built up over many years of eating refined foods. This fast cleanses the colon of pesticides, preservatives, dyes, drug residue, and parasites imbedded in the thick, hard lining. The colon actually has the ability to manufacture certain vitamins, and it continues to absorb nutrients until food waste is expelled from the body. But the mucous lining can inhibit and prevent this absorption and the manufacture of vitamins and minerals. Some people carry as much as 60 pounds of this waste material in the colon. Take a minimum of one or two internal baths per day, depending upon the matter being released. If the matter is not expelled during this fast, wait for 7 or 8 weeks and repeat the process; few people need to do this fast more than twice to get results. Your last internal bath should be an acidophilus cleanse or implant (see chapter 7), to replace the beneficial bacteria in the large intestine.

ENDING YOUR FAST

Upon completion of the fast, your first solid food should be oranges, or carrots that have been lightly steamed. Stick to raw and steamed vegetables and fruits with simple dressings for the first day or two. Then begin adding grains, nuts and seeds, dairy, and fish as desired. It is important to keep rice dishes in the diet after cleansing fasts. Rice promotes excellent digestion and tones the entire digestive system. Reestablishing the beneficial bacteria in the colon is very important. Flavor plain yogurt with apple juice, cinnamon and nutmeg, or vanilla extract. Rejuvelac (wheatberry juice), Kombucha tea, or liquid acidophilus will achieve the same effect. If you prefer, buy the powerful encapsulated acidophilus cultures for sale in the refrigerated section of natural foods stores. Continue to take acidophilus therapy for at least 30 days after completing your fast. Use $^1/_2$ cup of plain yogurt or liquid acidophilus in the morning on an empty stomach and $^1/_2$ cup at night before bed, or take acidophilus capsules as directed on the bottle. Capsules are preferable to powder forms as the gelatin shell protects the bacteria strains from oxygenation.

Important Note: The ingredients in soft drinks destroy the beneficial flora in the colon, as do drugs and foods adulterated with refined white sugar, flour, and preservatives. It takes up to 1 year to reestablish beneficial bacteria in the colon. Therefore, it is best to avoid overuse of junk foods and drugs, particularly antibiotics, after your fast.

The following cleanse is taken from *Good Health Through Special Diets* by Hannah Kroeger.[3]

🍃 SIMPLE COLON CLEANSE

Add ingredients to a container. Cover container with lid and shake to blend. Drink slowly, but do not let drink thicken too long. Then drink more fluids like herb tea or water, so that you have a total fluid intake of 16 ounces. Do this 5 times a day: 7 A.M.-10 A.M.-1 P.M.-4 P.M. and 7 P.M. Before

INGREDIENTS	AMOUNT
apple juice	½ C.
water (approximate)	⅓ C.
psyllium combination or psyllium hulls	1 heaping tsp.
liquid bentonite (Sonne's No.7)	2 or 3 T.

retiring, take an enema to eliminate all the waste from the colon so that you may sleep soundly. On the fourth or fifth day, besides long ropes of waste (mucous lining), you will lose dark matter, which is a sign that you may start adding food to your diet—such as raw and steamed vegetables and fruits. Reestablish friendly bacteria with acidophilus or yogurt and go on a good natural diet.

The following recipe is from Dr. Bernard Jensen and is a pleasant addition if desired. Dr. Jensen's book, *Tissue Cleansing Through Bowel Management*,[4] contains some of the most extensive information on the subject of intestinal health and is recommended reading for those who wish to learn more regarding this area of health. If you cannot find this book at your natural foods store, ask to have it ordered or write to Dr. Bernard Jensen to order a copy. See Sources.

🍃 REVITALIZING BROTH

This broth is very easy to digest and is good for the colon while fasting.

Choose 5 or 6 of these non-gas–forming vegetables: beets, carrots, potato peelings, celery, parsley, okra, chayote pear, or any squash. (Do not use

INGREDIENTS	AMOUNT
cut-up vegetables	1 C.
pure water	2 C.
organic soybean milk	2 T.

any of the sulfur vegetables: cabbage, cauliflower, broccoli, or onion.)

Simmer all ingredients except the soy milk for 3 to 5 minutes over a very low flame. This will break down the fiber and release enzymes. Strain the broth before use; then add soy milk.

Colon Care Notes: When traveling in other countries, you may find that the toilet is often a hole in the floor and you have to squat. This is the normal eliminating position, the one in which all of our internal organs are held in proper position. Modern toilets place great strain on the eliminative organs due to the unnatural sitting position. To rectify, place your feet on a small stepping stool while sitting on the toilet or raise your arms above your head to relieve the stress of a sitting position.

Besides eating a wide variety of fresh raw foods, ancient cultures usually included fermented food in their daily diet. The Eskimos have their special way of making sauerkraut, the south sea islanders have fermented taro flour called *poi*. In Africa a special drink is fermented from millet. These people enjoy exceptional health and vitality. Fermented foods are rich in lactic acid, which controls unfriendly bacteria in the digestive tract. Soured foods such as buttermilk, plain yogurt, and black sourdough bread are among the many fermented foods to enjoy.

ALOE-PAPAYA JUICE FOR DIGESTION

Combine equal parts of aloe vera juice with papaya puree concentrate to create a delicious drink that will sooth the stomach lining and stimulate the whole digestive process very effectively. Aloe vera and papaya in combination is one of the best and most delicious drinks to indulge oneself after completing any fast. The digestion is noticeably improved in a very short time.

PARASITE PATROL

We all have parasites in one form or another; they are a physical fact of life. Some types do not adversely affect health, but other types can cause a wide range of health problems. These parasites are evasive creatures that can remain in the body for a lifetime and go undetected in medical testing due to their nocturnal nature. They become most active around the time of a full moon. The body's protective mechanism is to build cysts and tumors around them to protect against irritation; this also hinders parasite detection and removal.

A parasite is any organism that lives in or on—at the expense of—another organism. No organ of the body is immune to invasion, including the brain, eyes, blood, heart, and liver. They thrive in the digestive organs from the stomach to the colon, where they love to nest and lay their many eggs. If problem parasites become numerous enough—or in the case of a tapeworm, large enough—they can block the colon, greatly inhibiting its function.

There are over a thousand different kinds of parasites that can enter the body through ingestion of raw contaminated foods and water (such as drinking from mountain streams and rivers), through open wounds, or from animals and insects. Wind and air currents can distribute microscopic eggs. Some are picked up from the soil in hot tropical places and burrow through the skin of bare feet. Pets and other animals can pass on parasites, and sexual activity can also transmit parasites from one person to another.

A recent study by the World Health Organization concludes that intestinal worms, round worms, whip worms, and hookworms afflict about 1.4 billion people worldwide. Regular deworming is an effective tool in preventing blood loss and anemia in the 400 million school-age children around the world who are infected. An antiparasite drug, given 3 times a year, prevents the loss of about a quarter liter of blood per child.

PHYSICAL MANIFESTATIONS

The most corrosive parasites thrive best in the nutrient-deficient and toxic-laden body. If you are undernourished or your immune system is weak, it is easy for parasites to take over. Worms and parasites live in a degenerative environment; they are very toxic to the system, and it is known that many degenerative and incurable diseases are parasite-related. Some physical manifestations of parasitic conditions include uneasiness, chronic fatigue, body odor (including feet), teeth grinding at night, hormone imbalance, anemia, AIDS, anal itching, voracious appetite, weight loss, mental depression, bowel infection, ulceration of intestinal wall, abdominal pain, diarrhea; shortness of breath and other lung inflammations such as asthma; painful and enlarged liver; nausea, dizziness, insomnia, acne, constipation, intestinal bleeding, low hemoglobin levels, tonsillitis, appendicitis, colitis, tumorlike masses, prostate problems, seizures, convulsions, fits, excess mucus, multiple sclerosis, and leprosy. The skin of infected people is often pale and sickly look-ing with a gray cast. A victim may have dull eyes that lack sparkle. It is no wonder that parasites are hard to diagnose. The symptoms listed can apply to many other conditions.

PREVENTIVE MEASURES

The good news is that no worm or parasite can exist out of its environment. Therefore, if you change your inner environment through cleansings and eating good foods, "your" parasites cannot exist. Preventive measures include steering clear of raw beef and fish. It is best to avoid pork altogether, since tests show that pork parasites remain alive after the meat has been cooked to a char. Keeping the diet free of junk foods will definitely dis-courage parasites. Fruits, vegetables, and meats can be soaked in the food baths (p. 133) before storage or preparation to decontaminate them. Pets and animals should be treated yearly to prevent a ping-pong effect. Be careful of salad bars in restaurants and avoid cheeses that have been aged a long time. Wash your hands after working in the soil and after using the rest room. Avoid swallowing mucus from your throat, practice safe sex, and keep your colon clean.

Everyone should cleanse twice a year for problem parasites. The cleansing fast for the large intestine along with parasite patrol are the two most effective practices we can utilize to rid ourselves of parasites. It is amazing how the years fall away after cleansing and the rosy glow of the skin, sparkling eyes, and the wonderful feeling of well-being replace the aspects of decline.

ANTHELMINTICS

Anthelmintics are medicines that destroy or aid in expelling worms and parasites from the body. Some of the best and most efficient of these are pinkroot, wormseed, wormwood, male fern, pumpkin seeds, castor oil, pomegranate rind, garlic, black walnut, diatomaceous earth, and the color yellow.

Pinkroot is the most efficient remedy for the many types of roundworms. Pinworms, a type of roundworm, often afflict children. They are found in the appendix and are associated with both acute and chronic inflammation of that bowel section. Another type nests in the lungs during a stage of the larva and, if numerous enough, causes shortness of breath and other lung inflammations, as well as intestinal blockage and irritations, diarrhea, constipation, jaundice, and appendicitis. Taking drugs often drives the worms into the liver and bile duct.

Given in moderate quantities, pinkroot produces only transient unpleasant effects. It does not destroy but simply narcotizes the worm. It should be used in connection with an active aid for expelling the worms such as castor oil or senna tea and yellow-charged water.

American settlers learned of pinkroot's efficacy from the Native Americans, but it fell into disuse in the early 1900s. It was so popular that dealers secretly adulterated it or substituted with other plants. In actual practice, the fresh root is preferred; it should not be used if more than two years old. The twenty-third edition of the *Dispensatory of the United States* lists the prescribed dose of powdered root for an adult as 4 or 8 grams taken each morning and evening for several days. This sequence is then to be followed by a strong laxative. Keep the diet light and simple while taking the herb. It is best used during a full moon.

FROZEN CASTOR OIL CAPSULES

Frozen castor oil capsules are a good remedy to help loosen and flush out the nesting areas of the worms during and after your chosen treatment for parasite patrol. The frozen capsules melt near or in the colon, acting as a cathartic and removing the black mold nests and eggs. Because of individual differences in size and weight, more or less may be needed for the best results. Make the capsules by filling gelatin or vegicaps with a good brand of castor oil and freezing them. Take 3 to 6 capsules of the frozen oil in the morning before breakfast and again just before retiring. Start with a small amount and increase if needed. It is advisable to limit activities so that you are near a rest room when using castor oil.

Note: Vegicaps are made from all-vegetable, naturally occurring plant cellulose ingredients. They contain no preservatives, are faster dissolving, and neutral to the digestive system. See Sources.

DR. JOHN CHRISTOPHER'S FORMULAS

The late Dr. John Christopher was a master herbalist who wrote many books on healing. His formulas are available for order. See Sources.

❧ WORMWOOD AND MOLASSES FAST

This is a famous formula of Dr. Christopher's for eliminating parasites. Wormwood is an extremely bitter remedy but is an excellent anthelmintic. The formula is particularly effective against

INGREDIENTS	AMOUNT
powdered wormwood	*1 tsp.*
blackstrap molasses	*1 T.*

roundworms. In Germany, this herb is very popular as a tea when mixed with honey and lemon. To enhance the effect of this formula, use as many raw onion and garlic dishes in the diet as possible.

TIME: Surrounding full moon
TIME FRAME: 3 to 6 days

Combine the two ingredients well and take, morning and night, on an empty stomach. The parasites are attracted to the sweet molasses and are tricked into ingesting the toxic wormwood. On the third day, use a strong laxative herb such as senna or frozen castor oil capsules to clear the system. Keep the diet light and simple while taking the herbs.

Note: Keep figs and raw almonds along with cayenne pepper, pineapple, and fresh raw onion and garlic in the diet to discourage parasites.

❧ PARASITE TEA AND HONEY FAST

TIME: Good anytime, best during full moon
TIME FRAME: 1 to 3 days

Wormwood tea is poisonous to worms in the system. The tea is bitter, but the honey is sweet and draws the worms out; maple syrup can be substituted for the honey if preferred.

Boil 2 pints of pure water and add 6 tablespoons wormwood; boil another 10 minutes and strain. Sweeten with honey or maple syrup. Drink the sweet tea throughout the day, $1/2$ to 1 cup at a time as desired, until about 8 P.M. Then make a standard medicinal laxative tea (chapter 7); drink 1 or 2 cups before bedtime. In the morning, take an enema therapy treatment, using the recipe for Garlic Cleanser (p. 190) as the enema bag solution. Repeat this whole process for up to 3 days or more to cleanse the body of parasites. Castor oil and lemon should also be used to clear the digestive tract after the treatment (refer to chapter 7).

AMERICAN WORMSEED

Native Americans knew that the Jerusalem oak was the best vermifuge (worm-killer) in Nature. Other names for this herb are the American wormseed, jesuit's tea, and goosefoot. Dr. John Christopher thought very highly of this old Native American remedy. American wormseed is contained in his VF liquid herbal formula, which is blended with many other herbs. See Sources.

TAPEWORMS

Tapeworms are among the oldest problem parasites afflicting the human race. The fish, pork, and beef tapeworms are considered the most dangerous. While some people lose weight, most become overweight when tapeworms are present in the body. Tapeworms can raise blood sugar levels, causing a misdiagnosis of diabetes, and they may cause anemia, seizures, or epilepsy. Passage of portions of the worm is a positive sign of inhabitation, along with other general symptoms such as abdominal pain, ravenous hunger, movement in the bowels, and distention of bowels with gas. Other signs are alternate constipation and diarrhea, headaches, nightsweats, deafness, blindness, heartburn, palpitation, itching about the anus, and tickling of the nose. Very often there are no symptoms except for the passage of portions of the worm and its eggs. The general symptoms may also continue for a time after the worm is expelled.

Tapeworm therapy is only successful when the whole worm has been expelled. If the tiny scolex (head) remains with its hooks imbedded in the tissue, the entire worm will grow back. If the head of the tapeworm digs too far into the intestinal wall, the injuries can be infected with bacteria and lead to ulceration of the intestinal wall. Therefore, it is advisable to do several treatments, 1 or 2 months apart, to ensure thorough results. If intestinal ulceration is suspected, use the aloe vera and flaxseed healing waters in enema or colon therapy, and also take them in the form of teas and juices.

THE FISH TAPEWORM

The fish tapeworm is the largest parasite that can grow in the digestive tract, reaching up to 40 feet or more. It is acquired by eating raw or undercooked fish that contain the larvae. The worm can often produce more than 1,000,000 eggs per day and can live for 20 years or more if unchecked. This tapeworm generally produces few symptoms aside from anemia or colon blockage.

The Food and Drug Administration has issued an advisory recommending that fish served raw, marinated, or partially cooked should be blast-frozen to 31 degrees F or below for 15 hours, or frozen by regular means to 10 degrees F or below for 7 days. Raw fish dishes include sushi, sashimi, seviche, gravlax, pickled herring, lomi, lomi salmon, and cold-smoked fish. There are also partially cooked fillets.

In addition to tapeworm larva in raw fish dishes, other potentially infective worms include roundworms or nematodes and two types of flukes. Therefore, freezing fish as described in the FDA advisory seems the most practical safeguard against parasites for consumers who wish to eat partially cooked fish.

THE BEEF TAPEWORM

The beef tapeworm is the second largest tapeworm, averaging 13 to 39 feet in length. It occurs in people who often eat raw or rare beef. Poisonous substances produced by this worm can cause convulsions and fits, fatigue, nausea, weakness, dizziness, or other symptoms. If beef is well-cooked, it is cleared of parasitic and bacterial contamination. (However, well-cooked meats of any kind are much more difficult to digest than rare, and they contain no dietary fiber. Therefore, be sure to include plenty of vegetables and salads if meats are consumed.)

THE PORK TAPEWORM

The adult pork tapeworm can live more than 25 years in the body and cause problems such as verminous epilepsy or seizures, due to the larvae and cysts of the pork tapeworm in the brain. The parasites that exist in pork can be difficult to kill. This is the reason many cultures do not use pork in the diet even though, traditionally, pork is served well-cooked.

OTHER TAPEWORMS

The 1½-inch-long dwarf tapeworm is the most common in the southern United States.

The dog tapeworm is passed on when infected animals lick your face or hands, or it can be spread from animal hair to the hands. Wash hands and face well after contact with pets and do not allow them to eat from household bowls and plates.

🌿 PINEAPPLE FAST FOR THE LUNGS
TIME: Surrounding full moon
TIME FRAME: 3 to 10 days

Incomplete digestion and poor nutrition, along with free radicals from rancid fats, can result in particles of matter that gradually close the "pores" of the lungs. The lungs then lose their elasticity. Pineapple and pineapple juice are good for lung problems, high blood pressure, tumors, and expelling intestinal worms. The enzyme bromelin in pineapple destroys tapeworms and most other worms—it even dissolves the protective coating at the cyst stage of life and the larvae inside.

Recipe: Eat fresh pineapple, as much as you like, for 3 days. Wormwood and ginger tea can be added during this fast along with figs, raw almonds, and whole pumpkin seeds if desired. Take a strong laxative tea or the frozen castor oil capsules the morning or night of the third day, and during the rest of the fast to help expel the matter. Use the Garlic or Flaxseed Cleanser (chapter 7) for enema or colon therapy treatments. They are excellent ways to cleanse the large intestine at the end of your fast for parasites. Yellow-Charged Water (see pp. 132, 179) is also recommended.

DIATOMACIOUS EARTH
Diatomacious earth is the remains of microscopic sea life from ancient oceans. It has been used successfully to eliminate parasites from the body; take 3 capsules twice a day. Check your natural foods store for this product.

BLACK WALNUT
Black walnut can be used to rid the body of many different types of parasites, along with the fungus and mold they live on. When their food supply is destroyed, parasites die and leave the body. An easy way to take black walnut is in tincture form, 20 to 25 drops on an empty stomach, morning and night. Add the tincture to herbal teas or fresh (not canned) pineapple juice or water. Black walnut hull powder can be taken (2–3 capsules) twice a day, morning and night, followed by the standard recipe for black walnut leaf herbal tea. Use laxative teas, castor oil, and internal baths to clear the system by the third day.

PUMPKIN SEEDS

The seeds of the common pumpkin have been used since ancient times to rid the body of tapeworms, with the advantage of being perfectly harmless to the system. Pumpkin seeds are also efficient for killing roundworms. The active principle is in the acrid and resinous seed envelope (not the hull) surrounding the embryo. A few days before taking herbs for tapeworms, eat foods such as raw onion and garlic, pickles and salted fish to loosen the grip of the worm.

 PUMPKIN SEED TEA
   TIME: Surrounding full moon
   TIME FRAME: 3 to 6 days

   Crush 2 ounces raw whole pumpkin seeds in a blender or mortar with a little pure water. Boil 4 cups water and pour over the crushed seeds. Allow to steep 15 to 20 minutes. Strain and drink 1 to 2 cupfuls each day, morning and night, on an empty stomach. In addition, chew 1 or 2 ounces of crushed pumpkin seeds. Eat lightly and simply. At the end of 3 days, the frozen castor oil or laxative teas and the internal bath therapies are useful to thoroughly cleanse the matter from your system.

 GARLIC AND ONION WATER FAST
   TIME: Good anytime, best during full moon
   TIME FRAME: 3 to 4 days

   I once knew a man who ate raw onion like most people eat apples. This fast will appeal to those lovers of onion and garlic who also desire to rid the body of parasites. The recipe will surely kill and expel the worms.

INGREDIENTS	AMOUNT
onion	*1*
garlic clove	*$^1/_2$ to 1*
pure water	*4 C.*

   DAYS 1 THROUGH 4:
   Put onion and garlic through a juicer and mix the juice with the pure water. If you do not have a juicer, cut up the onion and garlic and soak them overnight in the water. In the morning, squeeze all the juice out of the onion and the garlic solids through cheesecloth or cotton gauze, and drink remaining liquid. Drink

$^1/_2$ cup at a time throughout the day, and eat nothing. Extra beverages can be taken in the form of plain water with peppermint and parsley juice or ginger and wormwood tea.

In the morning of day 3, take 1 tablespoon castor oil. At night, take an enema therapy treatment, using the recipe for Garlic Cleanser as the enema bag solution.

THE COLOR YELLOW

Light and color have been used for healing throughout history with convincing and impressive results. Records taken from the pyramids reveal the use of colors for healing among the ancient Egyptians. Their system appears to have been highly advanced and to have given excellent results.

Dr. Edwin Babbitt wrote *The Principles of Light and Color* in the late nineteenth century, which became the first major contribution on the healing properties of color in modern times. Colonel Dinshah Pshadi Ghadalis also studied and wrote about color in the early twentieth century. The "readings" of Edgar Cayce provide additional evidence of the many healing qualities of color.

Einstein wrote that "all forms of matter are light waves in motion." All colors represent the energy of light waves in motion, vibrating at distinct and measurable rates. The divine science of color healing is a miracle of simplicity; it is not a fad or an illusion. It has been proven that color stimulates chemical action. By the application of color to our bodies, we introduce a natural energy that, among other healing effects, can help to eliminate waste and congestion. Color therapy has yielded superior results; it has played a role in repairing virtually every form of damage due to injury or sickness.

Applying the color yellow to fight parasites in the body is one example of the use of color therapy. Yellow benefits the body by strengthening and stimulating the organs—particularly the large intestine. According to Dr. Babbitt, applying the color yellow "has relieved cases of chronic constipation after the best known drugs had been tried in vain." Water charged with the sun's rays through yellow glass has been proven to be an absolute and unfailing cathartic; in small doses, a gentle laxative; and in all cases, exhilarating for the spirits. Worms and insects shy away from yellow, which destroys worms, driving them out of the body. Bug lights are colored yellow to keep insects away.

If we examine some of the foods used to treat parasitic conditions in the body, we see that they have a dominant yellow frequency; for example, there are pineapple, pumpkin seeds, castor oil, senna, prunes, egg yolk, and Epsom salts. (These are also laxative in their effect on the system.)

APPLYING YELLOW LIGHT

Placing a yellow lightbulb in a lamp and holding it 2 to 5 feet from the body for a maximum of 1 hour at a time, with 2-hour rest intervals in between, is the general procedure for using yellow light (or other colors) therapy. It is more effective if you are nude and in a reclining or sitting position during the light treatment. Other lights in the room will not affect the results, unless they are very bright or the room is flooded with bright sunlight. The best timing for applying yellow light therapy for parasites is on the days preceding and following a full moon, and particularly the night of the full moon. Treatments should be taken 2 hours or more after a meal is eaten.

For those with severe constipation, Dr. Babbitt suggests taking 2 to 4 tablespoons of **yellow-charged water** before each meal and every hour afterward. To make the treatment water, a yellow glass bottle or clear glass bottle wrapped in yellow cellophane is filled with pure water and left in the sunlight for at least 8 hours to a maximum of 24 hours. It must be used within 18 hours, after which it loses its charge. Yellow-charged water is an excellent addition to any parasite treatment, especially if one prefers not to take other laxative formulas, such as senna tea or castor oil.

FOOD BATHS

A little extra time spent treating the foods you eat with the following food cleansing procedures is well worth the effort. Fruits and vegetables will keep much longer. The wilted ones will return to fresh crispness. The flavors of both fruits and vegetables will be greatly enhanced, tasting like they have just been taken from the garden. Meats and eggs, as well as vegetables and fruits, will be cleansed of dangerous sprays, harmful additives, radiation, bacteria, fungus, metallic, and parasitic contamination, to a great extent. The breakdown of the soil, use of chemical sprays, radiation of foods, and processing of foods with preservatives and dyes have greatly contributed to the deteriorating health of the human race. Those who have their own gardens and can regulate the type of contamination have a greater degree of protection than others who depend upon the commercial markets for their vegetables. The dangers from contaminated foods are greater than most of us realize, but they are well-known to research scientists. It is up to the individual to be vigilant about the foods eaten—how they are grown and how they are prepared—to ensure health and well-being. This depends largely upon understanding what constitutes nutritious food and what constitutes poison for the body.

The following food cleansing baths were originally developed and tested for 10 years at Sierra State University School of Nutrition. These concepts were adopted by Dr. Hazel Parcells and utilized as part of the Parcells System of Scientific Living for more than

30 years in her research. Dr. Parcells continued her work until well over the age of 100. See Sources.

BATH #1

It is Dr. Parcells' suggestion that this bath be used first if you suspect that your food has been irradiated. Irradiation leaves foods devoid of the electromagnetic energy essential for nutrition. This simple bath is used to remove radiation.

INGREDIENTS	AMOUNT
baking soda	1 T.
pure water	1 gallon

🍃 BAKING SODA SOAK

Dissolve the baking soda in the water of a large tub. See chart on this page for soaking times.

BATH #2

This special bath eliminates bacteria and poisons from foods, keeps them fresh for long periods of time, and improves overall flavor.

INGREDIENTS	AMOUNT
Clorox (Clorox bleach only)	1/2 tsp.
pure water	1 gallon

🍃 CLOROX SOAK

Dissolve the Clorox in the water of a large tub. See chart on this page for soaking times.

SOAKING TIME CHART: Group the food to be treated separately as shown. Do not soak ground meats; frozen meats and fish can remain in the Clorox bath until thawed.

leafy vegetables	10 to 15 minutes
root vegetables	15 to 30 minutes
thin-skinned berries	10 to 15 minutes
heavy-skinned fruits	15 to 30 minutes
eggs	20 to 30 minutes
meats, per pound (thawed)	5 to 10 minutes

After soaking, remove foods from Clorox bath and place in a freshwater bath for 5 to 10 minutes. Let the food drain well before refrigeration. If the foods are treated with the baths as part of your marketing day—before you put them away—time is saved by not having to wash them for preparation. The foods remain fresh much longer.

1. Wash hands before and after handling raw meat, chicken, fish, vegetables, and fruits, to prevent contamination.
2. A hard plastic cutting board is preferable to the wooden type because wood is porous and contaminating spores can seep into the board. Keep separate cutting boards for meats and vegetables. Wash them after each use in a mild solution of 1 tablespoon Clorox to 1 gallon of water.
3. Wash utensils thoroughly after cutting meats and before using them to prepare vegetables and other foods.

PETS AND FARM ANIMALS

Those who live and work with and around animals are vulnerable to more parasitic exposure than those who do not. A precaution that will be invaluable to the health of both you and your pet is to simply add garlic and onion juice to the drinking water of the animals. Cayenne pepper is known by farmers as a dewormer for their animals. These methods save a fortune on veterinarian bills and antibiotics for the animals. See Sources.

CAYENNE FOR PEOPLE

Cayenne pepper is recognized for its many health benefits and is used as an ingredient in many herbal formulas. The genus *Capsicum annum* includes red and green chilies, cayenne, paprika, and bell peppers. Cayenne originated in Central and South America where it was extensively used by the natives to cure many diseases including diarrhea and cramps. Cayenne benefits the heart and circulation, preventing heart attacks and strokes, as well as colds, flu, diminished vitality, headaches, indigestion, depression, and arthritis. As a tonic, use $1/4$ teaspoon 3 times daily. Vegicaps or gelatin capsules are helpful if the hot flavor of cayenne is difficult to take by itself. Cayenne pepper taken with goldenseal is a specific for colds and flu. Pack the hot and bitter herbs in the capsules; take 2 of each with lemon juice and water sweetened with maple syrup or honey. Repeat up to 3 times daily.

Cayenne powder or tincture can be rubbed on toothaches, swellings, and inflammations. A remedy for arthritis pain is to rub a little cayenne tincture over the inflamed joint and wrap a red flannel cloth around it.

PLANTAIN MAGNET

When a little cayenne is combined with plantain and applied as a poultice, it has remarkable powers to draw out any foreign object embedded in the flesh.

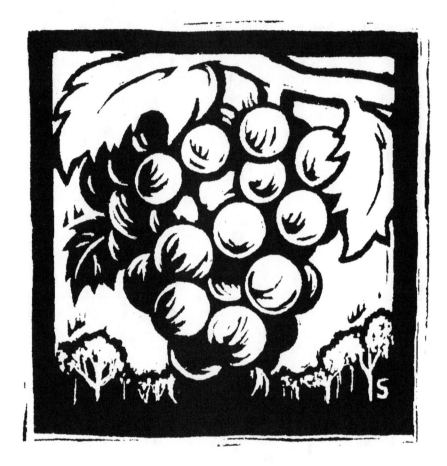

THE DOCTOR OF THE FUTURE WILL GIVE NO MEDICINES, BUT
WILL INTEREST THE PATIENTS IN CARE OF THE HUMAN FRAME,
IN DIET, AND IN THE CAUSES AND PREVENTION OF DISEASE.

—ATTRIBUTED TO THOMAS EDISON

AUTUMNTIDE FARE

THE BEST AUTUMN FOODS

The bounty of autumn rivals summer in abundance and beauty. The days are cooler, and we feel the intuitive urge to enjoy the rich, compact foods of fall. Allow extra time for storing and preserving foods from the garden for winter. Gather your herbs and be sure to include garlic. This is the time to plant new garlic for next summer. The fresh black and green figs that are available this time of year are not only excellent autumn fare, but they add beautiful color to any meal you make now. Fresh wild mushrooms are also nutritious fall fare.

BENEFICIAL AUTUMN FOODS

ORGANS: Lungs, large intestine
TIME: September 24 through December 20
COLOR: White
FRUITS: Apple, pear, persimmon, dates, raisins, grapes, fresh figs, pomegranate, and watermelon. VEGETABLES: Dark leafy greens, roots, carrots, onion, winter squash, leeks, ginger, garlic, brussels sprouts, kale, sweet potatoes, yams, collard greens, cauliflower, broccoli, and lettuce. HERBS: Shepherd's purse, coltsfoot, thyme, plantain, and horsetail. LEGUMES: Garbanzo beans and kidney beans. GRAINS: Brown rice, oats, barley, and wheat germ. DAIRY: Plain yogurt. MEATS AND EGGS: Fish, poultry, and egg yolks.

🍂 ULTIMATE AUTUMN OATMEAL

The addition of cloves, cinnamon, or nutmeg to oatmeal improves digestion, increases circulation, and is effective in warming the body in the chill of autumn. Oatmeal not only contains beneficial vitamins and minerals, but the bran has the highest protein content of all grains. Oats increase stamina and warmth, which makes them excellent cold weather fare. I like to use steel cut oats in this hearty recipe that will satisfy your hunger well past breakfast. Do not drink citrus juices with oatmeal; apple juice and herbal teas are better choices.

INGREDIENTS	AMOUNT
pure water	2¹/₂ C.
cloves (ground)	¹/₄ tsp.
cinnamon or nutmeg (ground)	1 tsp.
currants or raisins (organic)	¹/₃ C.
steel cut oats	³/₄ C.
oat bran	¹/₃ C.
shelled walnuts	¹/₃ C.
maple syrup (optional)	3 T.
organic half and half (optional)	¹/₃ C.

In a glass or stainless-steel saucepan, bring the water, spices, and currants to a boil. Add the oats, oat bran, and walnuts and stir for 1 minute. Turn off the heat and cover the pot tightly. Allow to stand 20 minutes, then stir. Enjoy as is or embellish with syrup and cream, a sprinkle of nutmeg, or toasted walnuts for a special occasion. Serves 2.

🍂 GARLIC SESAME GINGER DRESSING

All of the elements necessary to stimulate and help restore the lungs and large intestine during the autumn season are contained in this special dressing recipe. Enjoy it on salad greens or toss it with steamed vegetables and use it for vegetable marinades.

In a jar or wide-mouth bottle, combine the oils, herbs, and spices. In a small blender jar or measuring cup, blend the miso, sesame seed, mustard, and juices. Add this mixture to the oil and shake together.

INGREDIENTS	AMOUNT
olive or canola oil	¹/₃ C.
flaxseed or sesame seed oil	¹/₄ C.
fresh garlic cloves (minced)	2 or 3
fresh gingerroot (minced)	2¹/₂ tsp.
thyme (dried)	1¹/₂ tsp.
cumin and turmeric (powdered)	1 tsp. each
white miso paste	2 T.
white sesame seed	2 T.
prepared mustard	2 T.
apple juice	2 T.
aloe vera juice or gel	¹/₄ C.

Allow the flavors to meld before serving, and keep refrigerated. Makes 1¹/₄ cups.

DREW'S BAKED PUMPKINS WITH JIM'S ONION SAUCE

Baby sugar pumpkins are the novel centerpiece for this pleasing dish. It is fun to give each person a small pumpkin to carve and clean. Collect the pumpkin seeds to spread on a cookie sheet for a quick roasting. Enjoy them as a warm appetizer while the pumpkins are baking. This is simple cooking at its best—a dish created in honor of my father, Jim, and my brother, Drew.

INGREDIENTS	AMOUNT
baby sugar pumpkins	4
fresh rosemary sprigs	4
large yellow onion (quartered)	1
paprika	1 tsp.
vegetable broth	1¼ C.
kuzu root powder	1 T.
salted butter (organic)	4 T.
sherry	1½ tsp.
dark green mixed salad greens	5 C.

Carve a hole in the top of each pumpkin large enough to reach in. Remove the seeds with your hand and the remaining stringy pulp with a spoon. Place the pumpkins on a cookie sheet and put a sprig of rosemary and ¼ piece of peeled onion in each. Put the lids back on and bake the pumpkins at 350 degrees for 45 minutes or until tender. Spread the seeds on a cookie sheet (do not wash) and sprinkle lightly with sea salt. Bake them until crunchy and golden (15 minutes). Enjoy the seeds warm with a glass of red wine if desired. When the pumpkins are done, discard the rosemary sprigs and place the onions in a saucepan with the paprika and vegetable broth. Return pumpkins to the oven to keep warm. Dissolve the kuzu root powder in enough cold water to make a thin paste. Bring the onion broth to a boil and stir in the kusu paste until thickened. Add the butter and sherry; remove from heat. Cut each pumpkin in half and spoon the onion sauce into the center of each half. Serve with a dark leafy green salad and Garlic Sesame Ginger Dressing. Serves 4.

CURRY POTATO SALAD WITH KIDNEY BEANS

Kidney beans in a salad not only taste great, but they contain the essential fatty acid omega-3, important for our immune systems. This hearty potato salad, served with a green salad, is a meal in itself. Best served freshly made and at room temperature.

Wash, dice, and steam the potatoes until tender (do not peel). In the meantime, wash and dice the vegetables. Allow the potatoes to cool before cutting into bite-size pieces. Sprinkle the vinegar and Spike Shake evenly over

the potatoes and toss. Allow
to marinate 15 to 20 minutes.
Combine the raw vegetables,
herbs, potatoes, and kidney
beans with the Curry Dressing
below. Serves 8 to 10.

INGREDIENTS	AMOUNT
thin-skinned potatoes	8 C.
celery	3 C.
red onion	1½ C.
green pepper	1½ C.
fresh cilantro or parsley	¼ C.
kidney beans (cooked and drained)	2 C.
Curry Dressing (below)	
apple cider vinegar	¼ C.
Spike Shake (p. 41)	1 T.

❧ CURRY DRESSING

Boil the eggs for 3 minutes,
then immerse in cold water
until cooled. Separate yolks
from whites (discard whites)
and place yolks in a small
bowl; yolks should be runny.
Add remaining ingredients
and stir until combined.
Distribute dressing evenly
over potato salad, and toss.
Sprinkle the top with more
paprika.

INGREDIENTS	AMOUNT
egg yolks (soft boiled)	4
olive oil (rosemary flavored)	1 T.
Worcestershire sauce or tamari	1 tsp.
curry powder	2 tsp.
apple cider vinegar or lemon juice	1 T.
thyme or oregano	1 tsp.
cayenne pepper	to taste
paprika	½ tsp.
prepared mustard	1 T.
canola mayonnaise (cold-pressed)	¼ C.

❧ MICHAEL'S OCTOBER BIRTHDAY DINNER

This special dish is rich and colorful and has all the good attributes of a well-
combined meal. The beige, bell-shaped butternut or danish squash is the festive
centerpiece, so choose nicely shaped, medium-size squash, well suited for individual servings. (Acorn squash will also work nicely for this dish.)

Cut squash in half lengthwise, remove the seeds, and steam or bake at 350
degrees, seed side down, until tender (25–45 minutes). If you bake the squash,

place the potatoes in the oven with it (bake a dessert at the same time if you like). If you steam the squash, add the potatoes or brussels sprouts to the steamer. Slice the chard into bite-size pieces and steam lightly. In the meantime, gently melt the butter with the sherry and scallions, but do not

INGREDIENTS	AMOUNT
butternut or acorn squash	2 whole
new potatoes or brussels sprouts (halved)	8 to 12
red chard (chopped)	2 C.
organic butter	4 T.
sherry	2$^1/_2$ T.
scallions (diced)	$^1/_2$ C.
salad greens (mixed)	4 or 5 C.
fresh figs	12

boil. Fill centers of squash with a mixture of new potatoes and chard, then drizzle the butter sauce over the top of each. Place one squash half in center of plate and surround with mixed salad greens (Garlic Sesame Ginger or Kumari Curry would be excellent salad dressing choices.) Cut the figs in half and place them evenly around the rim of each plate (cut side up). Serve with wine or Mataji's Soothing Chai Tea and follow with dessert such as Baked Apples Marcel (p. 142). Serves 4.

🍂 MATAJI'S SOOTHING CHAI TEA

Chai teas and drinks originated in East Indian cuisine. They are so delicious that you will want to make extra to keep the goodness flowing. This drink goes well with almost any dish and is remarkably satisfying in place of coffee after a meal, as well as being good for digestion. Make this elegant drink in advance for guests and serve warm or cool with a sprinkle of spice.

INGREDIENTS	AMOUNT
pure water	2 C.
fresh peppermint leaves or	2 T.
dried peppermint leaves	1 T.
raw cow's milk or soy milk (organic)	1 qt.
cinnamon stick (whole)	1
cloves (ground)	$^1/_4$ tsp.
ginger (ground)	1 tsp.
cardamom (ground)	$^3/_4$ tsp.
black peppercorns (whole)	1 tsp.
sweetener (maple or	2 T. or to taste
brown rice syrup, or honey)	

Boil the water, remove from heat, add peppermint, and steep (covered) 20 minutes. In the meantime, simmer the milk and spices on low heat for 30 minutes. Strain and combine the peppermint tea with sweetener. Combine the spiced milk with the tea. Serve in small teacups or glasses, with a sprinkle of ground nutmeg, cloves, or cinnamon. Delightful! Serves 8.

🍂 BAKED APPLES MARCEL

Apples are considered a universal fruit because they complement everything. I used Yellow Delicious apples for this recipe, but any variety would work well with the rich date filling. This is a very special recipe that you will find elegant enough for any occasion.

INGREDIENTS	AMOUNT
apples (medium)	4
sherry or rum	1 T.
maple syrup	2 T.
brown rice syrup	2 T.
cinnamon	$1/2$ tsp.
mace	$1/4$ tsp.
medjool dates	3
raw almonds (shelled)	8
flaxseed (whole)	$4^1/_2$ tsp.
heavy cream, vanilla, nutmeg	garnish

Wash and core the apples, making sure the bottoms are intact to hold the stuffing. Trim the top of each apple to make a flat surface; do not peel apples. In a small bowl, combine the sherry or rum, syrups, and spices. Pit the dates and mince them into the syrup mixture. In a seed or nut grinder, grind the almonds and flaxseed to a fine meal and combine with the date mixture. Stuff each apple with the date filling. Mound the remaining filling on the top surface of the apples. Place them in a covered baking dish and bake at 325 degrees for about 20 minutes or until just tender. Remove from the oven but keep the lid on so they stay warm until you serve them. I like to thinly cover individual plates with heavy cream flavored with vanilla, and place an apple on top. Alternatives to using heavy cream are evaporated skim milk, sweetened oat milk, or nut milks with banana puree. Sprinkle with nutmeg and serve. Serves 4.

Note: A simple way to prepare the cream is to add 1 teaspoon vanilla extract or rum to $1/2$ -pint carton of cream, close tightly, and shake vigorously for 30 seconds. This gives it just the right consistency. Mix apple juice with cream to lower fat content if desired.

BROWN RICE

In the Orient, rice has been identified with God for thousands of years. It has also been the principal food of most oriental peoples during these centuries. It has had an interesting and checkered history in the rest of the world. For instance, rice became a status symbol in feudal Japan after it was introduced as the spoils of a small border skirmish between a Chinese warlord and a Japanese shogun. In 1326 Osma I, founder of the Ottoman Empire, declared rice to be a profane food, insisting that its consumption led to indolence, venery, and prurient behavior. As a consequence, rice fields were burned, and cooked rice in any form whatsoever was banished from Turkish kitchens for more than century. (Though contraband rice was often eaten on the sly.) Rice was introduced to the United States in the mid-1700s. Today it is grown in many southern and southwestern states.

A special property of rice is that it can be stored indefinitely without any chemical preservatives or refrigeration. Natural, whole unpolished brown rice contains all the minerals, vitamins, proteins, and lipids (organic compounds that make up fats) necessary to human nutrition. All rice is brown in its natural condition. It goes through a complex transformation process that strips the kernel from the husk, bran, and germ to achieve pristine and polished whiteness—leaving only the endosperm and very little else in the way of nutritional fiber. More than 7,000 varieties of rice are grown around the world. In the United States, the ones most conspicuously consumed are long-grain and medium-grain white rices.

❧ BOOK CLERK'S DELIGHT: ROASTED BROWN RICE AND NORI ROLLUPS

Roasting brown rice in a dry iron skillet (no oil) brings out a delicate nutty flavor. Small amounts of spices, seeds, and herbs add interesting flavors to the rice and are good for digestion. This simple recipe was inspired by a young clerk whom I often encountered on trips to the used-book store.

INGREDIENTS	AMOUNT
brown rice	2 C.
cumin (powder)	2 tsp.
pure water (boiling)	4 C.
sesame oil	1 or 2 T.
nori seaweed sheets	4 to 6

Rinse the rice in cool water, then place it in a heated iron skillet. (Be careful! The water will splutter.) Roast the rice until lightly browned, then stir in the cumin. Stir for 1 or 2 minutes, then transfer rice to the pan of boiling water. Cover the pan loosely with a lid and simmer gently for about 40 minutes. The rice is done when all water is absorbed and the rice is tender. Stir in the sesame oil. Cut the nori sheets into 4 pieces each and roll cooked rice in as you go. The rice rolls can be dipped in tamari soy sauce with wasabi (horseradish powder) if desired. Serves 4 to 6.

HOLIDAY BROWN RICE SALAD WITH FENNEL

Oriental people have long felt that natural brown rice is Nature's almost perfect food because it offers a treasure chest of nourishment. Brown rice contains 8 of the 11 essential amino acids, plus B complex vitamins, and minerals such as phosphorus and potassium. For those who are troubled with faulty digestion, rice is helpful; it assists the hormones to produce amylopectin, which promotes speedy and more complete digestion.

INGREDIENTS	AMOUNT
organic brown rice	1½ C.
pure water	3 C.
fennel bulb	1 large
celery stalks	3 large
roasted red pepper	1 C.
apple	1 large
fresh cilantro	1 C.
or fresh parsley and basil	½ C. each
scallions or	4
shallots	½ C.
marinated soybeans (optional)	¾ C.

The addition of marinated soy beans to this salad makes a complete protein dish.

This salad is a good one to make for special gatherings, and it keeps well in the refrigerator for meals at home. Other rice varieties can replace the brown rice if preferred.

Rinse the rice and place in a saucepan with the water. Bring to a boil; reduce heat. Cover loosely and simmer gently for 35 to 45 minutes. In the meantime, wash and dice all remaining ingredients except soybeans. The finished rice should be steamy and tender with no water left. Remove from heat and cool before combining with vegetables, fruit, and herbs. This salad can be dressed with Kumari Curry Dressing (p. 42) or try the dressing below. Serves 10 to 12.

🍂 HOLIDAY SALAD DRESSING

Blend all ingredients, except the apple juice, until incorporated. Use apple juice to achieve desired consistency (dressing should not be too thin). Add to rice salad and combine well. Garnish salad with tiny lady apples and greens or red roses and greens if desired.

INGREDIENTS	AMOUNT
rose water	$^1/_8$ tsp.
organic red wine	$^1/_2$ C.
mayonnaise	$^1/_2$ C.
organic lemon (juice and zest)	1
prepared mustard	2 T.
dried thyme, mint, marjoram, tarragon, and dill	1 tsp. each
fennel or anise seed	2 tsp.
apple juice	(to thin)

🍂 MARINATED SOYBEANS

Marinated soybeans are a perfect "fast food" because they remain delicious for up to 3 months after preparation. They are used in salads, sautés, dips, and grain dishes, adding a tasty nutritional boost in an instant.

INGREDIENTS	AMOUNT
soybeans (organic)	2 to 4 C.
pure water	to cover
tamari (marinade)	

Soybeans contain omega-3 fatty acids, and when combined with grains such as brown rice, they make a complete protein. Do not discard the tamari marinade after the soybeans are gone; use it for cooking or for other marinades. It is important to choose organic soybeans; commercial varieties can be quite contaminated with chemicals.

Soak the soybeans in water overnight. Discard soaking water and cover with fresh water. Cook until tender, drain (save water for soup stock), and cool. (Cooking times vary from $1^1/_2$ hours in a pressure cooker to 3 hours in a saucepan.) Place soybeans in glass jar and completely cover with tamari (or shoyu) to marinate. Do not refrigerate. Use as desired.

Note: In ancient times, tamari was widely used in its natural form and highly prized as a fine seasoning, having much the same flavor as present-day best-grade Chinese soy sauce. Today, an increasing amount is made synthetically and sold under various Chinese brand names. It is not brewed or fermented but is prepared from hydrolyzed vegetable protein. Its flavor and coloring come from additives such as corn syrup and caramel, and it may contain preservatives. Naturally fermented Japanese shoyu, sold as tamari in the West, is preferred in preparing all dishes calling for soy sauce. This seasoning, made from soybeans, salt, and water, contains 6.9 percent protein and 18 percent salt. Tamari is less expensive if purchased in bulk at a natural foods store.

🍃 TURKEY CHILI

This quick and hearty stew for a cold day is a tasty way to use up leftover turkey. Fresh turkey tenderloin cut into bite-size pieces or ground is a good use of leftovers in this well-combined, fat-free, complete protein dish.

Add cubed or ground turkey meat to stew pot with beer, onion, chili powder, cumin, oregano, and cayenne. Simmer for 5 to 10 minutes. Add water and rice, and cover tightly. When rice is tender, add tomato sauce and reboil. Remove from heat and add garlic and vegetables. Cover tightly and allow to stand for 20 minutes before serving. Garnish with parsley and serve with a side salad. Serves 10 to 12.

INGREDIENTS	AMOUNT
turkey meat	$1^{1}/_{2}$ lbs.
bottled beer (good quality)	1 C.
yellow onion (diced)	3 C.
chili powder	3 T.
cumin and oregano	2 tsp. each
cayenne pepper	dash
pure water	$2^{1}/_{2}$ C.
basmati rice	1 C.
tomato sauce	3 C.
garlic cloves (minced)	3
carrot (diced)	1 C.
bell pepper (diced)	1 C.
parsley (minced)	garnish

🍃 VEGETARIAN CHILI BEAN STEW

This is a rich, satisfying dish containing complete protein. Kidney beans contain the outstanding essential fatty acid omega-3. The kidney bean formed an important part of the diets of North American Indian tribes. The addition of asafetida to the soaking water is important to help neutralize gas-forming complex sugars in bean dishes. Asafetida, called *hing* in Sanskrit, has warming, antispasmodic properties and is preferred over garlic in Asian countries because it leaves no strong odor on the breath. This herb is found at East Indian and natural foods markets.

Cover the beans with hot water and soak for 2 to 3 hours or overnight. Drain, rinse, and place in the stewing pot along with 6 cups water, asafetida, bay leaves, cinnamon stick, chili powder, and molasses. Bring to a boil, cover, and simmer 1 hour or until done. While the beans are cooking, rinse the rice and place in a separate pot with 4 cups water. Bring to a boil, cover, and simmer till tender (35–45 minutes). Dice the vegetables, reserving enough onion to garnish the chili. When the beans are tender, add the tomato sauce and reboil for 5 to 10 minutes. Remove from heat, stir in remaining ingredients, except rice and garnish, tightly cover the

INGREDIENTS	AMOUNT
kidney beans (dry)	2 C.
pure water	6 C.
asafetida (hing)	1/8 tsp.
bay leaves	3
cinnamon stick	1
chili powder	3 T.
molasses	3 T.
brown rice	2 C.
pure water	4 C.
celery	1 C.
carrot	1 C.
red or green pepper	1 C.
red or green onion	1 C.
mushroom tomato sauce	3 C.
cumin, marjoram, and sage	2 tsp. each
cayenne pepper or red chili flakes	to taste
cider vinegar or beer	2 T.
smoked tempeh or tofu (diced fine)	garnish

pot and allow to stand 20 minutes or more to meld flavors. Serve over brown rice, or grain of choice, and garnish with onion and tempeh or tofu. A green salad is the perfect companion for the spicy chili. Serves 6 to 8.

❧ NO CRUST PUMPKIN CUSTARD PIE

Classic and simple, visually elegant, and the first dessert that vanishes with lightning speed at dinner parties. Quite simply my favorite way to make pumpkin pie—without the crust!

Choose good-quality canned pumpkin or have a bit of fun making your own with a sugar pie pumpkin. Cut the top open and scoop out the seeds to save; these are a crunchy bonus not included with canned pumpkin. (Spread the seeds over a cookie sheet, sprinkle lightly with sea salt, and bake until crunchy, 10–15 minutes). Pierce pumpkin with a knife in several places and replace lid. Bake at 350 degrees until tender. Remove from oven. While the pumpkin is cooling, beat egg yolks in a clear glass baking casserole, add milk and remaining custard ingredients. Scoop out soft pumpkin and blend all together until creamy. Bake in casserole for 10 minutes at 450 degrees, then 40 minutes at 350 degrees or until set. Cool. Whip the cream to hold its shape and flavor it with rum or vanilla. Spread the cream in soft mounds to cover the top of the pie and sprinkle lightly with nutmeg. A large, nicely shaped piece of can-

INGREDIENTS	AMOUNT
organic pumpkin puree	3 C.
egg yolks	2
evaporated milk or oat milk	1 C.
buttermilk	1 C.
maple syrup	$^1/_3$ C.
molasses	$^1/_4$ C.
cinnamon	1 T.
ginger	$1^1/_2$ tsp.
powdered cloves	$^1/_4$ tsp.
TOPPING	
fresh heavy cream	2 C.
rum or vanilla	$1^1/_2$ tsp.
nutmeg	sprinkle
candied ginger	garnish

died ginger looks like a jewel placed in the center, or it is pretty if finely minced. The glass lid to fit the casserole is perfect to protect the finished pie, which should be kept cool until needed.

CHAPTER SIX

WINTER
RESTORATION

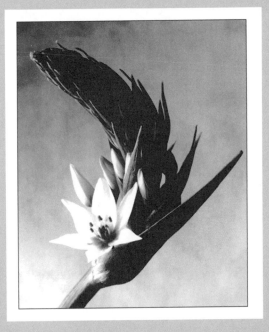

OUR TRADITIONS ARE OUR OWN, BUT OUR
ANCESTORS ARE THEIR ANCESTORS. WE ARE ALL
UNDER THE WINGS OF THE GREAT SPIRIT.[1]

—ALBERTO VILLOLDO

WINTER

Winter is the hardest season in which to cleanse, especially in the colder climates where more fuel is needed to keep the body warm. Winter is related to the element Water. Water is the essential liquid medium of your body through which all things pass. This fluid of life is important for functions such as the circulation of blood to carry heat and nourishment throughout the body; the lymphatic flow, which helps to process and eliminate wastes and provides your ability to fight off infections and other foreign agents; and the flow of urine, saliva, perspiration, tears, and sexual fluids. Sea water is almost identical in composition to blood plasma. Water is the circulatory system of Earth. Clouds, snow, lakes, rivers, streams, and the oceans are all part of this water circulation. Roughly 70 percent of Earth's surface is water, as is the human body.

The **bladder** and **kidneys**, which deal with the body's water, are the organs associated with the winter season. Interestingly, their condition can be read in the bones and in the hair on the head. The Water element is related to the emotions as well as to the sex organs and the sexual functions of the body. The bladder and kidneys are treated as one in a cleansing fast.

One of the chief functions of the kidneys is to rid the blood of excess water; they also work closely with the adrenal glands to oxygenate the system and regulate muscle tone.

THE BLADDER

The bladder is a thick, muscular organ in the pelvis that stores and eliminates urine received from the kidneys. As with other organs of the body, if it is not functioning well, the rest of the system is stressed. Tensions and held-in emotions can easily cause congestion in the pelvis area and can also lead to stiffness and neck or back pains. It is good to keep the energy in your back loose and flowing through stretching and freely expressing your feelings.

When difficulties arise in the bladder—such as infection—strong herbal teas may be used for relief: uva ursi, parsley root, juniper berries, marsh mallow root, cleavers, buchu, and gingerroot.

❀ THREE-CHARM TEA

The three herbs in this tea work like a charm to relieve bladder infection. It is also useful for blood in the urine. Tea made with uva ursi leaves is always cooled to room temperature before drinking it. This amount is enough for 2 days.

INGREDIENTS	AMOUNT
gingerroot	*1 T.*
pure water	*6 C.*
marsh mallow root	*1 T.*
uva ursi leaves	*4 T.*

Slice the gingerroot, if it is fresh, and simmer it in the water for 10 minutes. Turn off the heat and add the marsh mallow root and uva ursi leaves. Cover and let tea stand until it reaches room temperature. Take 3 cups daily.

The best herbs for the bladder are even more effective when combined with garlic to fight infection. Follow the Standard Medicinal Herbal Tea recipe (p. 213).

catnip	dandelion	kelp
taheebo	comfrey	echinacea
parsley	uva ursi	cornsilk
goldenseal	safflower	yarrow

✿ PINE NEEDLE TEA

The diced green needles (young or old) of pine trees can be used to make a tea that is rich in vitamins A and C.

INGREDIENTS	AMOUNT
pure water	*6 C.*
diced pine needles (green)	*1/3 C.*

Boil the water and remove from heat. Add the pine needles and let stand for 20 to 30 minutes before drinking.[2]

THE KIDNEYS

The kidneys, along with the liver, are the filters of the blood. There are two of these remarkable little organs—shaped like the bean named after them—which lie in the back just under the diaphragm. Their upper poles are covered by the last two or three ribs. The kidneys' main blood supply is arterial—the cleanest, reddest blood in the body. Snugly encased in a strong, inelastic capsule of fibrous tissue, they are embedded in a cushion of fat, thus protected from harm.

Three divisions are seen in a cross-section of a kidney. The first two divisions contain no sensory nerves and thus cannot register pain when impaired. In compensation, the pelvis is lined with cells richly supplied with sensory nerves that register pain from kidney stones or excessive acidity or alkalinity of the urine. (Also similarly equipped and sensitive are the ureter and the bladder.) A quality, balanced diet with plenty of water and adequate exercise are reliable preventive measures against kidney stones. Glomeruli are tiny, globelike filters in the kidneys, which become inflamed and eventually may be destroyed if the arterial blood is toxic. Toxicity is often the result of improper diet.

❀ WINTER KIDNEY CLEANSE

TIME: Winter
TIME FRAME: 7 to 10 days

Some signs of kidney trouble are stiffness in the neck, stiff and painful arms, back troubles, and fuzzy eyesight. In advanced distress, kidney troubles result in sore knees and swollen ankles.

INGREDIENTS	AMOUNT
celery leaves	*1 C.*
parsley	*1 C.*
distilled water	*1 1/2 qts.*

The right kidney filters mercury, copper, DDT, and arsenic-bound chemicals. The left kidney is sensitive to infections. Keep your kidneys healthy with this standard kidney cleanse. The Watermelon Seed Tea in Late Summer Restoration (p. 92) is also a good fast for the kidneys.

DAY 1: Fast with diluted fresh apple juice and distilled water. Mix 1/2 cup juice with 1/2 cup water. Drink the diluted juice whenever you are hungry. In between juices, drink 3 to 4 cups of the broth (above) from morning to night.

Wash and chop the celery and parsley leaves. Put them into a pot with the water and simmer for 20 minutes. Remove from heat and let stand for 15 minutes. Cool and strain before drinking.

DAYS 2 THROUGH 10: For breakfast, eat Bircher-Benner Muesli (p. 162) or plain yogurt with fresh fruit, and drink the celery and parsley broth or have chamomile and horsetail tea (refer to chapter 8). For lunch, have raw or cooked vegetables, salads with olive oil and lemon juice dressing, rice soup, barley soup, egg yolk, millet, baked potato, broiled fish, chicken, or turkey. Repeat breakfast drinks. Lunch should be the largest meal of the day. Choose 2 or 3 foods from the lunch menu and do not overeat. For supper, eat dark rye bread with organic butter only, vegetable soup, or grains such as brown rice and buckwheat (kasha), and herbal teas (as with breakfast) or diluted apple juice. Eat lightly for supper and do not have proteins of any kind. (Choose one starch per meal.)

Note: For those with kidney troubles, avoid alcohol, red meat, smoked meats, smoked or canned fish, and pork. Ready-made convenience foods are not good for the kidneys.

❀ BEET JUICE FAST FOR THE KIDNEYS
TIME: Winter
TIME FRAME: 5 days

Beet juice is excellent for the kidneys. It has been used to clean away gravel from the system. Take 1 tablespoon at a time, by itself, throughout the day.

DAY 1: Clean the digestive tract with the Epsom Salts Internal Bath (p. 181). At 3 P.M. begin taking 1 tablespoon fresh-pressed beet juice each hour up to 8 P.M. Drink distilled water in between when you are thirsty.

DAY 2: Continue taking 1 tablespoon fresh beet juice each hour from 8 A.M. to 8 P.M., drinking distilled water in between.

DAY 3: Choose a breakfast selection from the Winter Kidney Cleanse. At noon begin taking the beet juice each hour until 8 P.M. Do not have any other foods except distilled water in between.

DAY 4: Choose a breakfast and lunch selection from the Winter Kidney Cleanse. At 3 P.M. begin taking the beet juice only until 8 P.M. Drink distilled water only throughout the day.

DAY 5: Begin your day with 1 tablespoon beet juice in the morning. Wait 30 minutes, then choose breakfast, lunch, and dinner selections from the Winter Kidney Cleanse.

HERBS FOR THE KIDNEYS

In the Middle Ages, shave grass—otherwise known as horsetail—was most widely used for kidney problems. In old writings and stories, and in descriptions of herbs secretly kept in monasteries, shave grass was one of the top five herbs, along with chamomile, birch tree leaves, white nettle, and rosehips.

Follow the directions for Standard Medicinal Herbal Tea (p. 213), using the herbs and food listed on following page.

HEALING HERBS FOR RIGHT KIDNEY	HERBS FOR LEFT KIDNEY
pumpkin seed tea	cornsilk tea
watermelon seed tea	uva ursi tea
horsetail tea	fresh watermelon
male fern tea	female fern tea

When both kidneys are impaired, chamomile tea should be taken and continued for a month after all signs of illness are gone. The right kidney takes care of the waste material from below the middle of the body, and the left kidney from the upper body. It is true that men suffer a great deal more from kidney ailments of the right kidney, and women more from ailments of the left kidney.

Uva ursi and yarrow used in combination with other herbs give relief and promote healing of the entire urinary tract. Herbs for kidney stones include bitterroot, blue vervain, buckthorn, chaparral, horsetail, parsley, sage, and uva ursi.

❀ POTATO PEEL TEA

This valuable and effective solution for swollen ankles and legs is simple enough for anyone to make at home. It has been passed down from generation to generation. Cover potato

INGREDIENTS	AMOUNT
organic potato peelings	1 handful
pure water	2 C.

peelings with water. Simmer (low heat) for 15 minutes and strain. Use 2 tablespoons of the potato broth in 1 cup of water; drink 4 cups a day for 14 days.

❀ WINTER POTATO FAST FOR WEIGHT REDUCTION

Contrary to popular belief, the potato is not fattening. It is the added gravy, the sour cream, and the butter that boost the calorie count. It is natural to gain up to 10 pounds in winter to fortify the body in cold weather and keep it strong. However, if you desire to lose weight after the holiday season, or at the end of winter to prepare for spring, try a potato fast. This fast is also excellent for bowel trouble and good for a sensitive and irritated digestive tract. It provides nonirritating bulk.

In contrast to all other tubers, the potato provides complete protein. However, the nutritional value of a potato depends a great deal on the soil in which it is grown. Choose potatoes that are small to medium and feel heavy in the hand. Avoid those with such skin discoloration as green or dark brown spots (these can be poisonous). Do not use aluminum pots, pans, or foil when cooking potatoes. Potatoes are a good winter source of vitamins C and B₁ and the mineral potassium. Potato juice acts as an antacid, soothing the digestive tract.

TIME: Winter
TIME FRAME: 2 to 4 days

Morning, noon, and night, potatoes—baked, steamed, mashed, roasted, and juiced (not fried)—are eaten. Season the potatoes, if desired, with garlic (fresh and roasted), rosemary, nutmeg, dill, paprika, caraway, fennel, turmeric, cumin, chive, or mint. Juice raw potatoes and use the liquid when mashing steamed or baked potatoes. Try raw potato juice combined with herbal teas. Always leave the skins on the potato; they contain 75 percent of the mineral value. Utilize the different varieties of potato, but avoid all other foods. Eat only when you are hungry.

Good herbal teas to drink in between potato meals are corn silk (reduces fluid retention), burdock, nettle, yarrow, and dried or roasted dandelion root. All are good kidney and bladder herbs for winter. Drink the potato-peel tea (p. 154) for variety and in combination with herbal teas. Utilize the internal bath of your choice if desired.

THE ADRENAL GLANDS

The adrenal glands were long regarded as emergency glands—pouring out their internal secretions only when a person was confronted by a dangerous situation and had to resort to "fight or flight." Later, it was shown that adrenaline is so vital that humans cannot live for 4 seconds if it has been drained from the blood. An example is the sudden death that results from cyanide poisoning, which puts a stop to all oxidation in the body.

The chemical process of filtration of toxins through the kidneys depends upon oxidation, which is literally a process of burning. The adrenal secretions make oxidation possible. The body has extra depots for the manufacture and storage of adrenaline, such as the brain and the great nerve ganglia, the posterior pituitary, the sex glands, and scattered areas throughout the kidneys. This explains why some animals, and occasionally even humans, are able to live after removal of the adrenals. Another adrenal function is to regulate the strength of muscle tone; this includes the bowel muscle as well as the skeletal muscles. The adrenal glands lie against the upper poles of the kidneys, perched on them like caps.

❀ FATIGUE FAST FOR ADRENAL EXHAUSTION

We run out of energy when the adrenal glands do not provide us with enough cortisone or when we have maltreated this organ with junk foods. The following 1-day fast is a European folk remedy to help restore adrenal function.

1. Soak 3 tablespoons alfalfa seeds in 1 quart of water overnight; then bring to a boil and simmer 10 minutes.
2. Strain and drink as a breakfast beverage with a pinch of sea salt.
3. Drink the rest of the tea without salt throughout the day.
4. Blend 2 tablespoons sunflower seeds and 10 dates in 1 cup water, and eat slowly, chewing well. This restores energy beautifully. Foods good for the adrenal glands are vitamin C, egg yolks, and lecithin.

ADRENAL STRESS

A craving for salt is one sign of adrenal stress. When craving salt, feed the glands with juices and foods that are high in organic sodium. These include beets and beet greens, spinach, parsley, celery, and carrots. In addition, foods rich in pantothenic acid such as mushrooms, split peas, perch, pecans, soybeans, lightly cooked egg yolks, broccoli, cauliflower, kale, and lecithin stimulate the adrenal glands to produce hormones and increase output in response to stress. Antistress hormones are also produced in vitamin C rich foods, some of which include hot and sweet peppers, kale, parsley, broccoli, brussels sprouts, red cabbage, rose-hip tea, citrus fruits, and strawberries.

As for other nutrients that feed the adrenal glands, most fruits and vegetables are rich in potassium; magnesium is found in beet greens, spinach, and parsley; zinc is in gingerroot, parsley, and potatoes; and vitamin B_6 is in kale, spinach, and sweet peppers. Whey has the highest natural sodium content of any food. Sodium has the ability to dissolve calcium deposits around the joints, and whey is beneficial for the relief of arthritis since it dissolves calcium deposits, allowing the bloodstream to carry them out of the body.

The following juice recipes are rich in antistress nutrients. Juice ingredients and drink several 8-ounce to 10-ounce servings a day during stressful times to protect your body from the adverse effects.

❀ STRESS EXPRESS

INGREDIENTS	AMOUNT
carrots	4 to 6
celery (with leaves)	2 stalks
kale	2 leaves
parsley	$^1/_2$ C.
apple	$^1/_2$
fresh gingerroot	$^1/_2$ tsp.
whey powder	2 T.

❀ GARDEN MARY

INGREDIENTS	AMOUNT
tomatoes	2 or 3
green pepper	$^1/_4$
broccoli florets	3
spinach	$^1/_2$ C.
hot pepper sauce (Tabasco)	dash
or cayenne pepper	
whey powder	2 T.

❀ MIXED VEGGI

INGREDIENTS	AMOUNT
carrots	3 or 4
celery (with leaves)	2 stalks
beet	$^1/_2$
fresh mint	$^1/_2$ tsp.
whey powder	2 T.

❀ WINTER TISSUE CLEANSING

Oranges are a valuable winter food on our North American continent. They are full of vitamin C and are a good winter fasting food to discourage colds and cleanse the calcium deposits in the body. They strengthen the eyesight and immune system, and clear mucus from all bodily tissues.

INGREDIENTS	AMOUNT
orange juice (fresh squeezed)	³/₄ C.
lime juice (fresh squeezed)	¹/₄ C.
pure water	¹/₄ C.

TIME: Winter
TIME FRAME: 3 days

1. Make the juice as needed and drink 8-ounce portions throughout the day when hungry or thirsty. Have a minimum of 6 drinks per day.
2. Three times a day drink a warm herbal tea made from one of the following herbs: goldenseal leaf, comfrey, fenugreek, myrrh, echinacea, black walnut leaf, barberry, buchu, or catnip.
3. Utilize the internal bath of your choice, and take sweat baths or the Rosemary Bentonite Bath in chapter 7.

❀ LYMPH CLEANSE

The "tree-like" lymphatic system in the body contains twice as much liquid as in the blood vessels. Lymphatic flow helps process and eliminate wastes resulting from the heat and energy created in rebuilding worn-out tissues. The lymphatic system makes it possible to fight off infections and other foreign agents. When the lymph nodes become clogged with waste products, we feel pain. A good massage therapist who specializes in Lymphatic Pulsatilis Techniques will be able to assist with lymphatic congestion.

The following lymph cleanse is especially useful to help relieve the toxic burden on the lymph system. If you come down with a winter cold or flu, be sure to do a lymph cleanse!

1. Drink the following on an empty stomach: 1 quart distilled water mixed with 2 level teaspoons sea salt. Or use Epsom Salts Internal Bath (p. 181).

2. Stroke your skin with a skin brush, using single strokes toward your heart.

3. Grate a heaping handful of raw ginger, wrap it in cheese cloth, and immerse it in your hot bath.

4. Drink a cup of hot ginger tea (chapter 8) while bathing. Stay in the bath for a minimum of 20 minutes. Blue violet tea is also good for the lymphatic system.

5. Stay warm (wear a bathrobe, slippers, etc.) and go to bed.

6. Stay covered, warm, and sweating for 20 to 30 minutes or more.

7. Massage your body with equal parts olive and peanut oil combined with a few drops of peppermint or lavender, then take a cool soapy shower. (Optional: shower and skin brush again.)

8. Combine juices to make a total of 1 gallon. Use fresh pink grapefruit, oranges, and pineapples. Add 1 cup each of fresh lemon and lime juices to the gallon of juice. Fast on this for 2 days and drink plenty of distilled water.

ALUMINUM TOXICITY

There is no established function for aluminum in human nutrition, but it is used in many ways that filter into our foods. Aluminum weakens the living tissue of the alimentary canal—the digestive tube from the mouth to the rectum. Many of aluminum's harmful effects result from its destruction of vitamins and the displacement of the minerals in the foods we eat. Yet, it is used in the water purification process and the manufacture of cooking pots, foil, table salt, baking powder, deodorants, certain antacids, some processed cheeses, and as a bleaching agent to whiten flour.

Usually, most of the aluminum taken into the body is ultimately excreted, but excessive amounts cause symptoms of poisoning. These include constipation, colic, loss of appetite, nausea, skin ailments, twitching of the leg muscles, excessive perspiration, and loss of energy. Motor paralysis, areas of local numbness, gastrointestinal inflammation, and senile dementia are also linked to aluminum toxicity.

Adele Davis reports that magnesium can displace aluminum in the body, and that aluminum toxicity was relieved after taking magnesium supplements.[3]

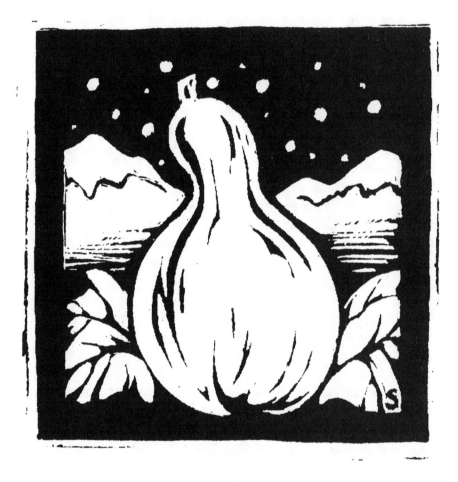

LIFT THE SELF UP BY THE SELF, AND DO NOT LET THE SELF DROOP DOWN. FOR THE SELF IS THE SELF'S ONLY FRIEND, AND THE SELF IS THE SELF'S ONLY FOE.

—AUTHOR UNKNOWN

WINTERTIDE FARE

THE BEST WINTER FOODS

The joy of winter eating depends upon our basic knowledge of autumn's bounty and our ability to preserve it, plus a little creativity. The best winter foods are designed by Nature to keep well and hold up throughout the cold winter months. Winter foods are fun! Yuletide is the time for mulled apple cider, wassail, and gingerbread. The New Year inspires dishes made with cabbage, potatoes, carrots, and black-eyed peas for good luck. "Imbolc," or Groundhog Day, calls for spicy, hot dishes made with garlic and chilies to help usher in the first green signs of spring! Winter foods are generally more building than cleansing. Eat more starches and proteins during the wintertime and search for those fruits and vegetables in season during the winter. Sweet root vegetables, onions, and citrus fruits, notably ruby red grapefruits (more vitamin C than white variety), are good winter foods, as are nuts and nut oils.

BENEFICIAL WINTER FOODS

ORGANS: Kidneys, bladder
TIME: December 21 through March 20
COLOR: Blue, black
FRUITS: Apples, cranberries, grapefruit, oranges, persimmon, pomegranate, and pineapple. VEGETABLES: Sturdy greens, kale, roots, celery, winter squash, pumpkin, sea vegetables—hijiki and kombu. HERBS: Rosemary, juniper, birch, and yarrow. GRAINS: Brown rice, buckwheat, and oats. LEGUMES: Soybeans, kidney beans, adzuki beans, and black-eyed peas. MEATS: Fish, poultry, game, and lamb.

❀ BIRCHER-BENNER MUESLI

Bircher-Benner, the famous international health spa of Switzerland, offers this satisfying breakfast cereal to patients as part of their daily healing diet. The qualities of this dish are said to be of great benefit to the kidneys.

INGREDIENTS	AMOUNT
rolled oats (organic)	4 T.
almonds (whole)	1 T.
pure water	³/₄ C.
heavy cream	4 T.
apples	3
honey	2 T.
lemon juice	2 tsp.

As a substitute for apples, you may use dried or seasonal fruits such as figs, cherries, prunes, and apricots, but do not use citrus fruits.

Soak the oats and almonds in water overnight, or soak in hot water until soft; the cereal will have a watery texture. To each serving, add 2 tablespoons of the thick cream and 1¹/₂ apples, finely grated. Add honey and lemon juice to your taste. Serves 2.

❀ WASSAIL

In cold weather, warm yourself with wassail, mulled apple cider, and herbal tea. The main ingredient in wassail is apples, which are sacred foods associated with many ancient deities. When eaten, the apples gave the gift of perpetual youth to the goddesses and gods.

INGREDIENTS	AMOUNT
fresh apple cider	2 qt.
cinnamon sticks	2
whole cloves	7
fresh gingerroot (sliced)	1 inch
nutmeg (whole)	1
lemon (sliced thin)	¹/₂
orange juice	1 C.
honey or maple syrup	to taste

In a glass or stainless steel saucepan, gently heat the apple cider, spices, ¹/₂ or ¹/₄ of the whole nutmeg, and lemon over low heat for 20 minutes, or until hot but not boiling. Remove from heat and let stand for 15 minutes. Add juice and honey or maple syrup to taste. Garnish each cup with a piece of cinnamon stick.

❀ EGGNOG CASHEW MILK WITH WHEY

Cashew nuts are high in protein but also high in calories. They are good body-builders for vitality and strong teeth and gums. They are best eaten raw—much easier to digest. This is a delicious, nourishing eggnog made without the cream.

INGREDIENTS	AMOUNT
raw cashew nuts (organic)	$^{1}/_{3}$ C.
pure water	$2^{1}/_{3}$ C.
egg yolk (soft boiled)	1
fresh orange or pineapple juice	$^{3}/_{4}$ C.
whey powder	1 T.
vanilla extract	$1^{1}/_{2}$ tsp.
mace	$^{1}/_{4}$ tsp.
honey or maple syrup	3 T. or to taste
nutmeg or cinnamon	garnish

Whey is a mild creamy liquid left over from cheesemaking. It has the highest content of natural sodium of any food. Arthritis sufferers benefit from whey's ability to dissolve calcium deposits around the joints. Whey helps feed the beneficial bacteria in your intestines, aids in reassimilation of nutrients, promotes regularity, and contains rich amounts of B complex vitamins for a youthful appearance.

In a blender, grind the nuts to a powder and then add the water. Blend the nut milk liquid with remaining ingredients and serve in cups garnished with freshly grated nutmeg or cinnamon. Serves 4 to 6.

WINTER SALADS

Adding sprouted seeds, beans, grains, and nuts to the diet will enliven many salads, stirred vegetable sautés, and even nut milks. Sprouts are highly nutritional and good complete protein foods. As most sprouts develop, their protein content increases; when they become green, chlorophyll and many vitamins are added and the protein ratio decreases.

Almost any seed or bean will sprout indoors during winter—some favorites are alfalfa, sunflower, radish, and onion. Alfalfa seeds can be mixed with other good sprouters such as lentil, mung, garbanzo, and adzuki beans. Grains, peas, and some nuts such as raw almonds will sprout. The almond carries more phosphorus and iron in a combination more easily assimilated than any other nut.

The seeds of amaranth—known to some gardeners as pigweed—are rich in high-quality protein, and both the seeds and the greens are loaded with calcium. Amaranth is one of the many edible weeds commonly discarded by home gardeners, who fail to appreciate their value.

Eating sprouted foods will infuse the vital energy of spring into your diet year-round. Sprouts are particularly valuable in the colder months when much vegetable life is in "hibernation" for the winter. For details on how to grow sprouts, see chapter 3.

❀ SPROUTED BEAN AND CHICKEN SALAD ADOBO

Adobo is a flavorful and simple way to prepare meat and vegetable dishes Philippine style. Winter foods should be comprised of more starches and proteins, essential for building and insulating the body. When meats are part of the diet, herbs like garlic and ginger should be used to offset the acids and purify the meat as much as possible. Too much meat in a diet breaks down friendly bacteria in the large intestine.

INGREDIENTS	AMOUNT
free-range chicken	1
sea salt and Spike Shake (p. 41)	2 tsp.
apple cider vinegar or wine vinegar	1/2 C.
bay leaves	2 to 3
whole peppercorns (black)	1 tsp.
garlic or fresh gingerroot (minced)	3 tsp.
assorted winter vegetables (diced)	6 C.
kuzu root starch	2 T.
tamari	1/3 C.
assorted bean sprouts	3 1/2 C.
scallions or red onion (sliced thin)	1/2 C.

Fowl, providing it has been organically fed, is the least harmful of meats. Choose a good-quality free-range bird. This dish can be cooked in the oven; at the same time roast beets for the beet and walnut salad following this recipe. Roasting should be done at a very low temperature to preserve food value—250 degrees for 20 minutes, then decrease to 125 degrees until done.

To reduce the hazards of possible contamination, soak the chicken in a solution of water and sea salt for 10 minutes, and rinse. Quarter the chicken and remove the skin, if desired, and sprinkle with Spike Shake. In a large stew pot, combine the vinegar, bay leaves, peppercorns, and garlic or ginger. Add the chicken and simmer for 20 minutes. Remove the peppercorns and bay leaves. Add the assorted winter vegetables and simmer until tender. Remove chicken and vegetables. Thicken the remaining liquid with kuzu root starch thinned with cold water. Remove from heat and stir in the tamari. Arrange the chicken and winter vegetables on a plate and drizzle with gravy. Garnish with the assorted fresh bean sprouts and onion.

❀ ROASTED BEET AND WALNUT SALAD

Beets are good food for the kidneys and bladder. They have blood-building powers and stimulate enzyme activity through the lymphatic system. Cooked beets should be eaten with their skins to benefit from all the vitamins and minerals.

INGREDIENTS	AMOUNT
roasted beets	3¹/₂ to 4 C.
apples	2 C.
freshly shelled walnuts	¹/₂ C.
green onion	¹/₂ C.
Italian parsley	¹/₄ C.
mint (dried)	2 tsp.
walnut oil	¹/₄ C.
fresh lemon or lime juice	2 T.
cinnamon	¹/₂ tsp.
honey	2 tsp.
tamari	2 tsp.
feta cheese	¹/₂ C.

Roast the beets until tender. Core and dice the apples, shell and chop the walnuts, and clean and chop the onion and parsley. Combine the mint, oil, lemon juice, cinnamon, honey, and tamari. Set aside. When the beets are cool enough to handle, dice them. Mix together in a bowl with cheese, apples, walnuts, green onion, and parsley. Drizzle dressing over, stir to coat. Serve at room temperature as a side salad.

❀ SPROUTED ESSENE BREAD

In general most commercially made breads, which contain hydrogenated oils, are congesting to the body. It is better to eat whole grain or stone-ground crackers—made without hydrogenated oils—than to eat too

INGREDIENTS	AMOUNT
hard durum wheat kernels	6 C.
pure water	10 C.
organic raisins (optional)	¹/₂ C.
almonds or walnuts (optional)	¹/₂ C.

much bread. This healthful recipe for sprouted bread is taken from the Dead Sea Scrolls, papyrus scrolls from the Essene religious community that date back to the second century. These expert bakers lived in self-sufficient collectives. Primarily vegetarians, their foods included various sprouted breads and wine. This technique produces a sweet, moist, cakelike bread without sugar, eggs, or oil.

In each of four 1-quart jars, place 1¹/₂ cups of wheat kernels and 2¹/₂ cups of water. Follow the sprouting instructions (p. 44). When the sprouts are about as long as the kernel, they are ready to use. A food processor or a meat grinder works well to grind the sprouts (2 cups at a time) into a sticky mass. Add the raisins or nuts as desired after the sprouts have been ground. Shape the dough into several round loaves (not too large). Place the loaves on a baking sheet, well oiled with grapeseed, canola, or olive oil. Cover the loaves and let them rest for 1 hour. Bake for 2 hours at 300 degrees or 4 hours at 250 degrees. (Baking the bread at low temperatures for longer periods of time preserves the freshness of the sprouted wheat. The ideal temperature would be around 100–115 degrees for about 8 hours.) Bake until the crust is browned and lightly toasted. Cool and refrigerate the finished bread. It keeps well, and is best if kept a day or two before serving.

❀ JAPANESE SOBA NOODLES WITH SESAME MISO SAUCE

Soba noodles contain up to 80 percent buckwheat, an excellent alternative to white pasta. Buckwheat is extremely nutritious, containing complete protein, vitamins, and minerals—especially manganese and magnesium. It is low in sodium and high in potassium. The rutin in buckwheat makes it a very important rejuvenating and age-retarding food. The sauce can be made with any nut or

INGREDIENTS	AMOUNT
buckwheat (soba) noodles	1 lb.
fresh gingerroot or lemon rind	2 T.
cooking stock or wine	1/4 C.
sesame butter (tahini) or peanut butter	1/4 C.
white or red miso paste	3 T.
cider vinegar	2 T.
tamari	1 T.
honey or maple syrup	1 tsp.
cilantro (chopped)	1/2 C.
green onion (chopped)	1/3 C.
chili flakes or paste (optional)	1/2 to 1 tsp.

seed butter. If you use peanut butter, make sure it is organic and without hydrogenated oils. Seed and nut butters should always be fresh.

Bring 2¹/₂ quarts of water to a rolling boil. Scatter the noodles slowly over the surface of the water and return to boil. Simmer uncovered for about 5 minutes or until tender—but not too soft. Strain and transfer to a large pot containing circulating cold water. Stir until cool, then drain well. Set aside. Grate the ginger (do not peel) or the lemon rind (organic). In a saucepan, add the ginger or lemon to the stock or wine, and heat until boiling. Simmer for 2 or 3 min-

utes, then add the sesame or nut butter; blend and remove from heat. Add the
remaining ingredients in the order given. Combine well. Toss the noodles and
the sauce together and serve with a green salad. Garnish with whole white
sesame seeds and cilantro if desired. Serves 4.

❀ ROSEMARY WALNUT PESTO

Rosemary is a wonderful
herb that grows throughout
the year, which makes it the
perfect candidate for a fresh
winter pesto. Beside being a
favorite pesto flavor, rosemary is high in easily assimilated calcium and thus is of
benefit to the entire nervous
system. Parsley leaves support the urinary tract and
relieve digestive weakness

INGREDIENTS	AMOUNT
olive oil	1/2 C.
flaxseed or hempseed oil (optional)	2 T.
garlic cloves (large)	2
cayenne pepper	pinch
walnuts (fresh-shelled)	1/2 C.
fresh rosemary leaves	1/2 C.
fresh parsley leaves	1 1/2 C.
freshly grated Parmesan cheese	1/3 C.
pecorino cheese	2 T.

and bronchial and lung congestion. Fresh pesto is a superb and elegant way to
keep fresh herbs in the diet, particularly in the winter flu season.

Process the first five ingredients in a blender or food processor. With the
machine running slowly, add the fresh herbs, then the cheeses. Process to the
desired consistency and allow to stand 5 minutes before serving. This pesto
sauce is good with vegetables, seafood, soba noodles, and lamb. Pesto will keep
refrigerated for 3 to 4 weeks, or it can be frozen for up to 6 months.

❀ ORANGE FLOWER WATER

Oranges are a valuable winter fruit. Orange flower water enhances the flavor of
water and lifts the spirit. Add 1 or 2 drops of orange oil to a quart of water for a
very pleasant and refreshing drink. Garnish with slices of fresh orange and lime.

❀ HOLIDAY HERBAL WINE

Fresh herbs, such as rosemary, and whole spices such as cloves, star anise, and
cinnamon sticks, are not only beautiful to behold but lend their aromatic
warmth to a decanter of wine; they also turn the wine into a comforting digestive

aid that helps to cleanse the
stomach. Choose a good
quality red or white wine
that is not too expensive. If
you have wine that is overly
tart or weak, herbs and
spices can be used to greatly
improve the flavor.

INGREDIENTS	AMOUNT
red or white wine	1 750ml bottle
fresh rosemary branches (4 to 6 inches)	1 to 3
whole cloves or star anise	3 to 4
whole cinnamon stick	1

Wash the rosemary and shake off the excess water. Put 1 or 2 branches in a
wide-mouthed, clean decanter. Pour the wine over the herb. A red wine may
need more rosemary than white wine. Add the spices and allow the flavors to
meld 30 minutes or longer before serving.

✤ NO-BAKE CAULIFLOWER CASSEROLE WITH PESTO CREAM

This no-bake casserole is simple
and elegant, a tasty dish that will
appeal to anyone who enjoys a
vitamin-rich vegetable and rice
dish. The pesto should be made
ahead to save time; use the
Rosemary Walnut Pesto recipe on
page 167. The fats used in this
dish are easily digestible and are
not overheated. Cream aids the
manufacture of lecithin necessary
to every body cell. It is also an
antiarthritic. The proper use of
good fats in cooking is the key to
keeping healthy fats in the diet.
Note: If organic rice is not used,
wash the rice well before roasting.

INGREDIENTS	AMOUNT
whole cumin seed	1 tsp.
black mustard seed	1 tsp.
fenugreek seed	2 tsp.
basmati rice	3/4 C.
brown rice	3/4 C.
pure water	3 C.
cauliflower	3 C.
red bell pepper	1 C.
yellow onion	1/2 C.
walnuts (optional)	1/4 C.
egg yolk (soft-boiled)	1
heavy cream	1/4 C.
Rosemary Walnut Pesto	3 or 4 T.

Dry roast the seeds and rice in a deep iron skillet over a medium flame until
lightly toasted and the spices become aromatic. Add the water to the rice mixture and bring to a boil. Reduce heat, cover loosely with a lid, and simmer until

water is absorbed and rice is tender (30–40 minutes). Clean and cut the vegetables into bite-size pieces as desired. When the rice is cooked, remove from heat and add the vegetables and nuts. Cover tightly and allow to stand for 20 minutes or more to gently steam the vegetables. Beat the egg yolk in a small bowl until smooth; incorporate the cream and Rosemary Walnut Pesto, stirring into a creamy sauce. Combine the sauce with the rice mixture. Serves 4.

❀ WARM WILD RICE SALAD WITH PEANUT SAUCE

Wild rice is not rice at all but an aquatic grass. It has twice as much protein as white rice. It is low in fat, high in the B complex vitamins, and contains higher amounts of amino acids and zinc than rice. Wild rice dishes are elegant enough for special gatherings. Try this salad with a vegetable soup, such as carrot-dill or squash, for a meal that will be a conversation piece. Experiment with the more exotic rices if they are available—Black Japonica or Wehani Indian rice. These have a nutty aroma and flavor that complement the peanut sauce. I always use good-quality organic peanut butter to make the peanut sauce. Peanut crops are highly contaminated with pesticides, and

INGREDIENTS	AMOUNT
wild rice	1 C.
brown rice	1 C.
pure water	6 C.
currants	3/4 C.
sherry	3 T.
green onion or cilantro	3/4 C.
mixed salad greens (dark leafy)	6 to 8 C.
creamy peanut butter (organic)	1/3 C.
apple cider or rice vinegar	2 T.
coconut milk (lowfat) or pineapple juice	1/4 C.
apple juice	1/4 C.
tamari	2 T.
fresh grated gingerroot	1 to 2 tsp.
thai chili paste	1 tsp.
(red pepper flakes or cayenne pepper can be used in place of thai chili paste according to taste)	

commercial peanut butter is hydrogenated. It is important to avoid all products containing hydrogenated oils.

Wash rices, and combine with water, bring to boil, cover and simmer until tender (40–50 minutes). Soak currants in sherry. Dice onion or chop cilantro. When rice is done, add currants, sherry, and onion or cilantro, and combine. Wash and dry salad greens and arrange on individual serving plates. Mix remaining ingredients together for the spicy peanut sauce, and set aside. Allow to stand for 5 to 10 minutes before serving. Mound rice in the center of the plate on top of the salad greens, top with peanut sauce and garnish. Red Miso Dressing (p. 96) is nice on a side salad with this dish. Serves 4 to 6.

❀ TIBBON'S PORTUGUESE BEANS

On the winter solstice of 1996, during a torrential downpour, we planted trees in San Francisco for Friends of the Urban Forest. My red rubber boots and yellow rain-coat were voted best-of-show. First prize, in the food category, clearly belonged to my friend Susan Tibbon for making the most delicious dark bean stew we ever tasted. After going to great lengths to get her recipe, I am happy that many others will now enjoy this rich dish. On that chilly and wet winter morning, it was perfect for breakfast, as well as lunch. If pink kidney beans, called "pink beans" at the natural

INGREDIENTS	AMOUNT
pink kidney beans	1 lb.
pure water	1/4 C.
large onion (chopped)	1
dark yeast extract (brewer's yeast)	1 T.
cinnamon	1 tsp.
ground cloves	1/2 tsp.
allspice	1/2 tsp.
ground cumin seeds	1 tsp.
Italian plum tomatoes, chopped	3 1/2 C.
blackstrap molasses	2 T.
dried hot red pepper	1 tsp.
fresh garlic (minced)	1 T.
tamari	1 T.
dark beer or stout (optional)	1/2 C.
apricot fruit conserve (optional)	1/2 C.

foods store, are not available, red kidney beans or black-eyed peas are good alternatives. This dish is more delicious if the spices are ground fresh.

Soak the beans in warm water for 8 hours or overnight; drain and rinse. Add 1/4 cup water to a soup pot and sauté the onion over moderate heat for 10 minutes; stir in the dark yeast extract. Add the cinnamon, cloves, allspice, and cumin to the onion mixture. Stir in the beans and enough water to cover the bean mixture. Bring to a boil, lower heat, and simmer covered for 1 1/2 hours or until just tender. Add the tomatoes, molasses, and red pepper. Uncover and simmer for 30 minutes more. Remove from heat and add the garlic, tamari, beer, and fruit, if desired. Cover tightly. Let stand for 15 minutes or more to allow flavors to meld. The sauce should be thick. Serves 8 to 10.

❀ WHITE WINTER SOLSTICE SUPPER

We first prepared this supper for a group of friends visiting from France. This meal, inspired by a recipe from the famous Greens restaurant in San Francisco, was unforgettable. If you have a food processor, the white winter vegetable casserole will be easy to prepare. If not, get a friend to help you peel and slice. It is worth it!

INGREDIENTS	AMOUNT
leeks (white parts only)	2 to 3
fennel bulb	1
small turnips or parsnips	4
celery root	1
baking potatoes (thick skinned)	6
organic butter or olive oil	2 T.
fresh garlic cloves (crushed)	1
sea salt	to season
red pepper	to season
fresh thyme (branches)	8 to 10
organic cream	1 C.
pure water	³/₄ C.
apple juice or sherry	¹/₄ C.
flaxseed	¹/₄ C.
pine nuts or brazil nuts	¹/₂ C.
sour cream and chives	garnish

Slice the leeks into ¹/₄-inch rounds or 2-inch strips, and wash them well. Quarter the fennel bulb, trim away core and slice lengthwise (¹/₄ inch thick). Peel turnips or parsnips and slice into ¹/₈-inch rounds. Cut away the gnarly surface of the celery root, then quarter and slice thinly. Heat oven to 350 degrees. Put scrubbed and salted baking potatoes in. Butter or oil the bottom of a baking dish, and rub with crushed garlic. Layer half of the vegetables in the dish, and season with salt, red pepper, and thyme leaves. Make a second layer with remaining veggies, and season. Combine the cream, water, and apple juice or sherry and add it to the dish. Dot the surface with remaining butter or oil. Cover the dish loosely and bake for 30 minutes. Grind the flaxseed and nuts together to make a fine powder. Sprinkle the surface of the gratin with the seed and nut mixture— return it to the oven for 25 minutes or until tender. Serve the gratin with the baked potatoes (split) garnished with sour cream and chives, if desired, and a green salad. Light the candles and enjoy! Serves 6.

✿ SHERRY CHESTNUT STUFFING

Chestnuts are low in calories and are a beneficial carbohydrate food rich in potassium and magnesium. They are good for heart problems and high blood pressure. They should always be eaten cooked or roasted because of their tannic acid content. Buckwheat groats, known as kasha in Russia, could be substituted for the millet in this recipe if desired.

INGREDIENTS	AMOUNT
chestnuts (roasted or boiled)	2 C.
millet	1 C.
Spike Shake (with kelp) (p. 41)	2 tsp.
sweet potato (medium)	1
dry sherry	1/4 C.
onion (chopped)	2 C.
celery stalks with leaves (chopped)	4
dried oregano, marjoram, and thyme	1 tsp. each
powdered ginger and cayenne pepper	1/8 tsp. each
organic butter or olive oil	1/3 C.
fresh sage leaves (1 T. dry)	3 T.
fresh rosemary leaves (1 1/2 tsp. dry)	1 T.

Much time can be saved if you buy preshelled and peeled chestnuts. If you have a good helper, shell, peel, and roast the chestnuts a day before you make the stuffing. With a sharp knife, cut an "X" on the round side of each chestnut. Put them in a pan, cover with water, and bring to a slow boil until the shells open. Remove from heat. Use a paring knife to remove the shells and skins. I think it is nice to leave them in various sizes, but if you buy whole shelled chestnuts, chop them roughly before roasting.

Roast the millet in a dry iron skillet, transfer it to a saucepan with 2 cups of water and Spike Shake with kelp; simmer until tender (15–20 minutes). Put the sweet potato through a juicer, add sherry, and set the juice aside. In a large skillet, sauté the onion, half of the celery, and the dried herbs and spices in the butter or oil for 5 minutes; stir in the chestnuts and cook for 7 more minutes. Add the remaining celery, millet, and fresh herbs. Heat thoroughly and remove from heat. Stir in the sweet potato juice and serve. Also good as poultry stuffing. Serves 4 to 6.

❀ HOPPIN' JOHN SOUP

In the southern United States, it is a bleak, black day that does not dawn with a pot of rice and black-eyed peas bubbling away on the cookfire. Black-eyed peas are a good storehouse of minerals, vitamins A and B, folic acid, pantothenic acid, and niacin. Traditionally, Hoppin' John is simmered with a ham bone, which I have omitted, but if you use a rich stock, this soup will have plenty of flavor.

INGREDIENTS	AMOUNT
rich chicken or vegetable stock	6 C.
pure water	8 C.
fresh rosemary branch	5-inch piece
bay leaf	1
garlic cloves	4 to 5
cayenne pepper	1/4 tsp.
yellow mustard powder	2 tsp.
dried black-eyed peas	2 1/4 C.
brown rice (short grain)	3/4 C.
celery (diced)	2 C.
fresh thyme	1/2 tsp.
yellow or green onion (chopped)	1/2 C.

Add to a large pot the stock, water, rosemary, bay leaf, garlic, cayenne, dry mustard, and black-eyed peas. Bring to a boil and reduce heat, simmering partially covered for 1 1/2 hours. Remove bay leaf and rosemary branch. Roast the brown rice in a dry iron skillet and cook separately with 2 cups pure water for 35 minutes or until tender. Remove from heat. Add the rice and remaining ingredients to the peas and cover tightly. Allow the flavors to meld for 20 to 30 minutes before serving. Serves 8 to 10.

❀ MAPLE AND THYME POACHED FIGS

Figs are rich in minerals that are easy to assimilate. They are mentioned in the most ancient of texts and are used today in many healing recipes. Red wine will give this dish a richer, less sweet flavor. Either way, it's very elegant. Fresh thyme enhances the richness of this dish.

INGREDIENTS	AMOUNT
fresh vanilla bean	3 inches
dry sherry or sauternes wine	3/4 C.
maple syrup	2 T.
fresh apple juice or cider	3/4 C.
dried calimyrna figs (sliced)	2 C.
fresh thyme leaves (minced)	1/2 tsp.
cold, plain vanilla yogurt	garnish
lemon zest	garnish

Slice open the vanilla bean and scrape out the seeds. Put the seeds and the bean in a saucepan with the liquids and figs. Simmer the mixture slowly, partially covered, for 10 minutes. Remove from heat and add the fresh thyme. Cover tightly to allow flavors to meld for 15 minutes. Remove the vanilla beans and skins. Serve the figs warm, with the syrup, in stemmed glasses topped with a yogurt and lemon zest garnish.

CHAPTER SEVEN

THE BATHS
INTERNAL AND EXTERNAL
WATER THERAPY

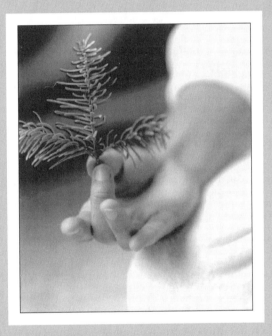

IN TIMES PAST, KNOWLEDGE OF THE BOWEL
WAS MORE WIDESPREAD AND PEOPLE WERE
TAUGHT HOW TO CARE FOR THE BOWEL.
KNOWING THE WAYS OF KEEPING THE BOWEL
HEALTHY, AND IN GOOD SHAPE IS THE BEST
WAY I KNOW TO KEEP AWAY FROM THE GRIP
OF DISEASE AND SICKNESS.[1]

—DR. BERNARD JENSEN

BATHS FOR THE INNER BODY

Good health is as much a function of how we eliminate waste from our bodies as what we actually ingest. If your system is upset during a cleansing diet or fast, it is because you are not having sufficient elimination. During any fast where colon therapy or an enema is not applied, you should have two, three, or more bowel movements a day. This may seem surprising if you are not eating solid food, but it is Nature's way of eliminating the waste it has loosened from the cells and organs in the body.

It is possible to fast without utilizing cleansing processes such as colon and enema therapies, and not all fasts require them. You should proceed at your own pace and comfort level. As you progress and, shall we say, "test the waters," you will find that the internal baths are not as difficult or threatening as imagined. It will then be possible for you to achieve greater degrees of body purification.

The colon completes the digestive process; it absorbs minerals, nutrients, and excess water from the digested residue of food we have eaten, and it discharges toxins and waste materials from the body. When the colon is clean and healthy, we experience a feeling of well-being. When it is congested with stagnant wastes, poisons back up in the system and pollute the inner environment. What develops is autointoxication—"self-poisoning"—in which toxins are reabsorbed and circulated through the cardiovascular system. Headaches, muscle soreness, fatigue, a sallow complexion, and other problems follow. In removing these toxins, which often are stored in intestinal crevices and in old fecal matter, we can greatly reduce the amount of toxicity in the body.

Working with internal baths in conjunction with a cleansing fast is a total restorative process for the body, mind, and spirit. The following recipes describe time-tested ways of bathing the body internally. There are various opinions as to which method to use during a particular cleansing fast or diet. Each of these methods has useful qualities. One may work better for a certain fast than another. Each fast suggested in *The Seasonal Detox Diet* is given with instructions regarding the internal bath that best facilitates the cleansing process of the body. After reviewing this chapter, you will know which internal baths you feel most comfortable with.

THE VALUE OF INTERNAL BATHS DURING FASTING

Generally there are two extreme attitudes regarding internal baths, which have been used for healing for centuries. On one hand, an individual is very accepting and comfortable with the idea and process. On the other hand, an individual is not at all comfortable with the process. The latter person may be mortified by the idea of actively cleansing the inner intestinal system—specifically the large intestine, or colon—through stimulation with various healing waters. I must emphasize, here, that the internal bath is an essential process in the healing arts. It is very important in the fasting process to relieve any nausea, headaches, or toxic symptoms that may occur, and to keep moving the poisons out of the system. All of the internal bath methods are also very helpful to use during illness—colds, or flu—to ease the toxic burden from the body and to promote quicker recovery.

HERBAL LAXATIVES

If you choose not to use colon or enema therapies, you should instead use a laxative herbal tea, which can be taken the night before you are to begin your fast. This will help the body to clear the way for the lighter foods you will be ingesting. Continue to take the teas first thing in the morning and last thing at night, until completion of the cleansing process.

Herbal laxative teas must not be overused, in general, as they can deplete the energy of the body. After a cleansing fast, proper elimination is very dependent upon proper diet. The teas should be prepared in stainless steel or glass vessels only. *Do not at any time use aluminum cookware, aluminum foil, tins, or cans, as these reduce the cleansing effects; aluminum contaminates both the foods and the body.*

Most of the brewed teas can be stored for up to 3 days, if kept cold, and can be gently reheated without boiling. Or you can drink the teas at room temperature. Actually, a good rule for drinking any beverage is to bring the liquid as close to body temperature as possible. This takes great strain off the digestive organs since liquids and foods in the stomach must be brought up or down to body temperature before digestion can begin.

❧ LICORICE ROOT TEA

Licorice root tea has a pleasant taste, and it is a good mild laxative. Licorice root can safely be added to detoxifying herbal formulas to alleviate the harsh, stimulating aspects of bitter herbs without interfering with the beneficial aspects asso-

INGREDIENTS	AMOUNT
pure water	*4 C.*
licorice root (broken)	*¼ C.*
apple, grape, or other fruit juices	*to taste*

ciated with their use. Licorice is considered one of the most important herbs of Chinese medicine and is frequently prescribed as part of Chinese herbal formulas.

Boil the water. Add the broken licorice root, and boil for 1 hour uncovered. Remove from the heat, cool, and strain. Drink ½ to 1 cup first thing in the morning. The tea is sweet and strong tasting; apple, grape, or other fruit juices may be added to dilute if desired.

❧ GENTLE LICORICE ROOT AND FLAXSEED TEA

Flaxseed is wonderfully soothing to the whole digestive system and is very good for internal irritations. In making this tea, the flaxseed should never be crushed because the healing mucilage is in the outer part of the kernel.

INGREDIENTS	AMOUNT
licorice root	3 T.
pure water	4 C.
flaxseed	3 T.
lemon juice and maple syrup	to taste

Boil the licorice root in water for 20 to 30 minutes, then pour it over the flaxseed, using a strainer to remove the root. Cover and let stand for 4 hours or overnight. Strain and add lemon juice and maple syrup if desired. Drink 1/2 to 1 cup morning and night.

❧ LAXATIVE BARLEY BREW

The East Indian tradition of Ayurveda is the oldest known formal systematic study of the human constitution. This brew is an Ayurvedic recipe inspired by directions in Nadkarni's *Indian Materia Medica*.[2] It needs a preparation time of overnight or a full day. Make this with organic barley only;

INGREDIENTS	AMOUNT
organic pearl barley	1/4 C.
organic figs	1/4 C.
licorice root	2 T.
organic raisins	1/4 C.
pure water	10 C.

otherwise this tea could concentrate toxins rather than relieving them.

Wash the barley well. Chop the figs and grind up the licorice root, if possible. Combine all ingredients with the water, cover and simmer slowly, until the liquid is reduced by half (about 8 hours, or overnight). Strain. Drink 1/2 cup morning and night.

❧ CARRIE'S BUCKTHORN BARK TEA

This special herbal tea that I prepare often is well received by guests in place of coffee any time of the day. Buckthorn bark is my favorite mild laxative herb for its beauty and because it is safe to use over an extended period of

INGREDIENTS	AMOUNT
pure water	6 C.
nettles, Oregon graperoot, and plantain	2 T. each
peppermint leaves	1 T.
buckthorn bark	2 T.

time. When combined with blood-purifying herbs, buckthorn bark helps to carry blood and liver toxins out of the body. It is even safe to use for ulcerative colitis and acute appendicitis. If you want to use buckthorn bark as a laxative during a fast, add 1 teaspoon bark to ½ cup cool water. Cover and let stand for 12 hours before drinking. To keep buckthorn bark in your diet, try the following recipe.

Bring water to a boil. Remove from heat and add all herbs except the buckthorn bark. Cover and let stand for 30 minutes and strain. Add the buckthorn bark, cover and let stand for an hour or two before serving. The tea may be reheated gently but reboiling it will destroy the healing qualities in the herbs. Other blood purifying herbs may be used in place of nettles, Oregon graperoot, or plantain. They include gota kola, marsh mallow, dong quai, ginseng, or elder flowers for colds and flu.

❧ CASTOR OIL

Castor oil, a medicinal rather than a cooking oil, has many therapeutic uses. It is an excellent way to clear the digestive tract, taking a modest ½ to 1 teaspoon before bed, or with a medicinal tea such as ginger, peppermint, or lemon water.

INGREDIENTS	AMOUNT
warm water	*½ C.*
lemon juice	*½ of lemon*
castor oil (begin with 1 T.)	*1 to 2 T.*

Taken internally, castor oil is one of the most reliable laxatives, and it is especially useful as a treatment for food poisoning. It is also taken along with anthelmintics to help dispel worms. It is not recommended for use during pregnancy.

Blend ingredients together and drink first thing in the morning. The lemon juice cuts the flavor of the oil nicely. More lemon and warm water, or peppermint tea, may be taken if desired. Castor oil can be taken in gelatin or vegetal capsules to eliminate the taste and feel of oil in the mouth. Try adding a drop of peppermint oil or extract to each capsule for aid in digestion.

❧ YELLOW-CHARGED WATER

People trained in color therapy know that a yellow frequency taken into the body stimulates the gastric juice and helps eliminate constipation. Utilizing the color yellow by charging distilled water with the sun's rays through yellow glass, and then drinking it, is found to be a gentle laxative and is exhilarating to the spirit. If a transparent yellow glass bottle is not available, wrap clear glass in yellow cellophane and set it outdoors exposed to the sun's rays—24 hours over the course of 2 or 3 days. Solarized water is taken in small amounts, 2 to 4 tablespoons, 3 times daily, or every hour for severe constipation. The yellow-charged water will lose its potency after 18 hours, so bottles should be prepared in rotation to complete any treatment. Yellow-charged water is excellent to use with treatments for parasites in the body because the color yellow is anthelmintic.

CASCARA SAGRADA AND GINGER TEA

Of all the plant medicines of North American Indians, cascara sagrada is the best known; it has become a favorite laxative throughout the world. In 1890 cascara bark was admitted to the *U.S. Pharmacopoeia*, and it remains an official medicine. It acts by irritating the bowel, inducing peristalsis. The *U.S. Dispensatory* adds, "It often appears to restore tone to the relaxed bowel and in this way produces a permanent beneficial effect." Those who benefit most from the action of cascara sagrada have atonic colons that balloon and are flaccid. Those with spastic colons should not use cascara sagrada often and, when doing so, should be sure to add mild herbs such as anise, fennel, licorice, and ginger to prevent cramping.

The bitter principle of cascara bark stimulates the secretions of the entire digestive system including the liver, gallbladder, stomach, and pancreas. It is one of the safest tonic laxative herbs known and is useful for colitis, hemorrhoids, and jaundice. Only bark that has been dried and aged for at least 1 year should be used.

❧ CASCARA SAGRADA TEA

Slice the gingerroot. Simmer in water for 30 minutes, remove from heat and cool. Add maple syrup and juice of 1 lemon.

When the ginger tea is cool enough to enjoy, take ¼ to 1 level teaspoonful of the powdered cascara bark in gelatin capsules with

INGREDIENTS	AMOUNT
gingerroot	2-inch piece
pure water	4 C.
maple syrup	¼ C.
lemon juice (fresh squeezed)	1 lemon
cascara bark	¼ to 1 level tsp.

the ginger tea. A tincture of cascara bark may also be added to the ginger tea in place of the powdered bark. Tinctures are highly concentrated herbal extracts that can be kept for long periods of time when preserved by alcohol. Use 10 to 30 drops in the ginger tea.

❧ ALOE VERA LEAF TEA

The dried powder of the aloe vera leaf is considered one of the best herbal laxatives to benefit the liver. However, it is a strong laxative herb and should be used with licorice root tea, or anise, fenugreek, or fennel seeds. The dried powder is bitter, but it can be taken in gelatin capsules with the licorice root or seed teas to prevent griping (cramping) in the intestines. Refer to the recipe for Licorice Root Tea (p. 177) if preferred, and use $^1/_2$ to 1 teaspoon aloe vera leaf powder to $^1/_2$ to 1 cup of the tea; or try the Seed Tea below if you prefer.

❧ SEED TEA

Using mortar and pestle, crush the anise and fennel seeds. Add to water in stainless steel or glass pot with fenugreek seed. Boil for 20 minutes. Steep for 10 to 20 minutes, strain, and take 1 cup with $^1/_2$ to 1 teaspoon powdered aloe vera leaf in gelatin capsules.

INGREDIENTS	AMOUNT
anise seed	1 T.
fennel seed	1 T.
pure water	2 C.
fenugreek seed	1 T.

❧ EPSOM SALTS INTERNAL BATH

Epsom salts are well utilized in times of fasting for both internal and external baths. These are a natural mineral salt containing magnesium sulfate, which is useful for restoring those with magnesium deficiency.

INGREDIENTS	AMOUNT
pure water	$^1/_4$ C.
Epsom salts	1 T.
orange juice	$^1/_4$ C.
fresh lemon juice (optional)	1 T.

Magnesium protects your nerves, much as calcium does, and it is especially effective at lowering blood cholesterol. Epsom salts are conveniently used as a short-term, saline laxative cleanser, but should not be taken for longer than 1 week. They should be avoided if you have a kidney disease. This drink is not salty tasting if taken with citrus juices.

Boil half of the water and pour it over the Epsom salts, stirring until clear. Add the remaining cool water and juices. Drink this solution when it has reached a comfortable temperature. Each $^1/_2$ hour after taking the salts, drink 6 to 8 ounces of water, herbal tea, or fresh diluted citrus juice to help flush out the digestive tract and keep the body well hydrated. A minimum of 3 quarts of liquid should be consumed; a maximum of 1 gallon is sufficient. The laxative effect of the salts will continue throughout the day. You will need to be near a rest room. No solid food should be consumed during the flushing process. Eating solid food will interrupt the cleansing of the intestinal tract. The oral laxatives are best utilized when you desire to clear the entire digestive tract in preparation for a fast.

RESTORATIVE LAXATIVE TEA COMBINATIONS

The following herbal combinations help to restore tone to a relaxed bowel and supply energy to the body. They clean mucus from the system, calm the stomach, fight infection, and clean and nourish the gastrointestinal tract, liver, and urinary tract.

1. Cascara sagrada, buckthorn, licorice root, capsicum, barberry, turkey rhubarb, couch grass, and red clover.
2. Dong quai, cascara sagrada, turkey rhubarb, goldenseal, capsicum, ginger, barberry, fennel, and red raspberry.

Use 1 tablespoon of each herb, from #1 or #2, combined with 5 cups pure water. Boil the roots for 10 to 15 minutes, turn off heat; add leaves and powders, cover and steep 10 to 15 minutes. Strain and drink 1/2 cup, 3 times a day. This is enough tea for 3 days. Keep refrigerated and do not reboil.

COLON THERAPY AND COLONIC IRRIGATION

A colon therapist is a licensed practitioner in the healing arts and may offer other health-enhancing services to your advantage, particularly during times of fasting. These may include various types of body massage to break up and facilitate the flow of toxins, iridology to help you understand the strengths and weaknesses of your body, acupuncture, and herbal therapy.

A colonic irrigation is an internal bath that helps cleanse the colon of poisons, gas, and accumulated matter. It involves safe, gentle infusion of purified warm waters into the colon, using no chemicals or drugs. A colonic irrigation simply bathes the colon, removing impactions from the colon walls, stimulating peristaltic action, and enhancing absorptive ability.

The use of colonic irrigation as a natural internal bath has been documented over thousands of years. The ancients used a hollow reed or bamboo tube to introduce water into the rectum by blowing into the tube. Or they would enter a river or lake to create the necessary pressure for the water to flow upward. Hindu scriptures tell of the practice and benefits of enemas and colonics. The Evers Papyrus, a medical document written about 1500 B.C., described the practice of colonic irrigation.

Today, a person receiving a colonic irrigation lies on a soft table near the temperature-controlled input tank. A special hygienic proctoscope is gently inserted into the rectum and the water flows into the colon via a small tube. There is a separate tube to drain the waste matter. As the water flows, the colon therapist gently massages the abdominal area to help release the contents in the colon. A steady stream of water flows gently in and out, stimulating the colon to recover its natural shape, tone, and peristaltic wave action. The person being treated is completely covered and kept warm during the procedure. The treatments can vary in length from 35 minutes to 60 minutes and are usually comfortable and relaxing. Cleansing the colon is easy when one is undergoing a fast because the soft foods and juices taken minimize bulk in the large intestine.

Many communities do not have therapists offering this service; if colonic irrigation is not available, the enema is useful. You may prefer to work with one or both, depending on where you live and how much time and money you wish to spend. To find a colon therapist, look in the phone book under colonic irrigations or inquire at your local natural foods store. Colonic treatments can vary greatly in their effects, due largely to the expertise of the colon therapist. Long and costly treatments are not necessary in most cases. Those individuals with known or suspected serious bowel problems, such as colitis or diverticulitis, need to approach colon therapy with extreme caution and consult with a naturopathic physician.

It is not surprising that Edgar Cayce, stressing the vital role of elimination in health, longevity, beauty, sexual vigor, and joy in living, gave this reply when asked about colonics: "When these are necessary, yes. For everyone should take an internal bath occasionally as well as an external one. They would all be better off if they would."[3] He suggested using a heaping teaspoon of table salt and a level teaspoon of baking soda—dissolved thoroughly—to each half gallon of water used for a colonic treatment. In the final bath, glycothymoline is used as an intestinal antiseptic to purify the system, in the proportions of a tablespoon to a quart of water. Glycothymoline is a mixture that, in former days, was inexpensive and available at most drug stores. Its main use was as a mouthwash. However, many of the larger chain drugstores do not carry it today. It can be found at natural foods stores, somewhat higher in price.

Do not hesitate to ask your colon therapist to add special ingredients to the purified waters. Prepare these and take them with you so that they may be easily added. Being able to discuss your needs with your health practitioner will allow him or her to participate with you on a deeper level of understanding regarding the restorative processes.

ENEMA THERAPY

Hippocrates and Galen were early advocates of enema therapy. The enema was often used by our grandmothers in their day. The advantages of using the enema are many. It is easy to work at your own pace at home, any time of day or evening. You can choose and prepare special recipes for the waters used internally. Massage techniques may be employed to ensure that the waters reach deep to cleanse the colon as thoroughly as possible. It is important to be patient with yourself and create as relaxing an environment as possible. Remain in a stress-free healing environment for the mind and body during the time you are working with enema therapy. It becomes a kind of healing ritual.

Begin by playing your favorite relaxing, soft music. Make the lighting soft also, so that there are no bright lights in your eyes. A candle or two will create a nice ambiance and will help to scent and purify the air and encourage deep breathing. Whether you are safely burning candles or using light bulbs, try dropping scented oils such as peppermint, eucalyptus, clove, pine, or menthol scent into the burning candle or onto the hot light bulb. This will diffuse the wonderful essence into the air and stimulate the lungs to draw deep breaths.

A great deal of elimination takes place through the lungs, by the way. When you take in a good deep breath, especially if you exhale it completely, forcing the residual air out of the lungs, you bring about a complete change of air. In breathing deeply, you not only bring oxygen down into the lower parts of the lungs, but you also help to speed the elimination of carbon dioxide, which is the end product of cell metabolism. Protein waste is also eliminated through the lungs in the form of carbon dioxide. The bloodstream picks up some of the acid waste and turns it into the gas, which is exchanged for oxygen in the lungs. When the breath is drawn in through the mouth and nostrils, it is destined to penetrate to the farthest cells. True, it may undergo many changes before it reaches its goal, but it will always carry an intention to travel to the furthest reaches of all extremities. When a constriction occurs in the pathways of these breaths of life, disease conditions develop quickly. Remember to breathe.

You should not find it difficult to purchase an enema bag at your local drugstore; if they do not carry it, ask to have it ordered for you. Choose and prepare the internal bath water you wish to use. Rinse the enema bag out with hot water and fill the bag with the solution, making sure the hose is clamped tightly closed. Then, to avoid air bubbles, release water through the hose (over a drain) until it pours out of the tube. Clamp the hose again, and find a roomy, comfortable place where you can lie down and where you can hang the bag 2 to 3 feet above you. A doorknob, a hook, or a rod will work well. If the bag is too high, it causes discomfort because the water runs too fast. A fluffy towel or rug to lie on is nice, or use old towels, or newspapers if you are inexperienced. Some individuals may even feel comfortable in the bathtub.

You will need to have simple oils such as olive, coconut, sweet almond, or any water-soluble oil (no petroleum jelly) close by to lubricate the short plastic rectal tip. The oils are also used to massage the abdominal area, and you may like to add scent to your oil for massage purposes.

A palm-size rubber ball or tennis ball is used to massage the colon in a counterclockwise direction. This helps to stimulate and loosen impacted matter and distributes the water throughout the colon, and is important to use especially during your fast for the large intestine.

Because there are many body types, each person should find the exact positioning that feels comfortable for the process. What works for some may not work for others. However, there are two basic positions that are generally successful. One simple rule to remember is that the water will enter the body on your left side (descending colon) via the rectum, move up across the body under the ribs (transverse colon), then down the right side of your body (ascending colon), left to right, or counterclockwise.

Lie on your back with your knees bent and feet flat on the floor. Insert the lubricated tip gently into the rectum, then turn on your left side in a knee-to-chest position, using your left arm as a pillow for your head. Depress the clamp and allow the water to flow in slowly. It is important to relax—take mental note and inventory of any tense muscles or feelings and let them go, as sometimes the tenseness will stop the water from flowing. Close your eyes if you like; allow the warm water to flow in only as long as you are comfortable with it. Then stop the flow of water, turn on your back with your knees bent—or your legs can be propped up on a wall—and gently massage the colon area from left to right (counterclockwise). You can use either your hands or the ball. If you are still comfortable, remain on your back and resume the flow of water, again only as long as you are comfortable with it. Then stop the flow of water and continue the massage, still lying on your back. Repeat this process while lying on your right side. The idea is to distribute the water throughout the colon as far as possible from left to right without discomfort.

When you feel the need to release the water, go to the bathroom and do so. Allow your body to guide you and progress at your own pace and comfort level. Expel the water solution if need be but avoid forcing the water and matter from the colon. Allow the colon to release the contents on its own. If the water does not release from the colon within 15 to 20 minutes, massaging the spinal column, twisting the torso, raising the arms to the ceiling and stretching upward, bending over, walking around, and moving the body in general, will all help to release it. Repeat this process, refilling the enema bag as many as six times, depending on the fast and matter being expelled. Six refills of the enema bag are about equal to one colon therapy treatment. Take breaks and rest in between.

Upon completion of this process, it is important to make sure as much of the internal bath water is expelled as possible. Be patient with your body. Once you have experienced how to work with this procedure, an enema becomes much simpler, and very quickly it all becomes second nature.

An alternate way to take an enema is to first lie on your left side, then on hands and knees, and finally lie on your right side. If you are still experiencing difficulty, lying on your back throughout the entire process with your legs propped against a wall will also work fine, as long as the abdominal area is massaged, following the shape of the colon from left to right. It is easy to tell how far the water has traveled because you can feel and hear it slosh around as you gently massage the area. Use circular motions for the massage to move the water through the abdomen. It is useful to study the illustration of the large intestine provided on page 187 for a better understanding of the specific anatomy of this area.

HEALING INTERNAL BATH WATERS

Planet Earth has many natural cleansing procedures for itself. Mother Nature has not forgotten us, either, and has provided a host of safe and wonderful things we can use in our cleansing procedures. Obtain the purest water and ingredients possible for these internal bath cleansing recipes. Always heat the water to lukewarm or use cool water near to body temperature before adding the ingredients. Some of the products used may only be available through a natural foods store, or ordering by mail may be necessary, depending on your location. If you have colon therapy, do not hesitate to prepare the following recipes to take with you so they may be easily used to further benefit your treatment.

❧ BASIC CLEANSER

Dissolve the salt and soda in warm, pure water. Omit salt and soda for the sixth quart of water used. Chlorophyll, acidophilus, or glycothymoline is a recommended addition for a rinse.

INGREDIENTS	AMOUNT
sea salt	*1 tsp.*
baking soda	*1 tsp.*
pure water (warm)	*4 C.*

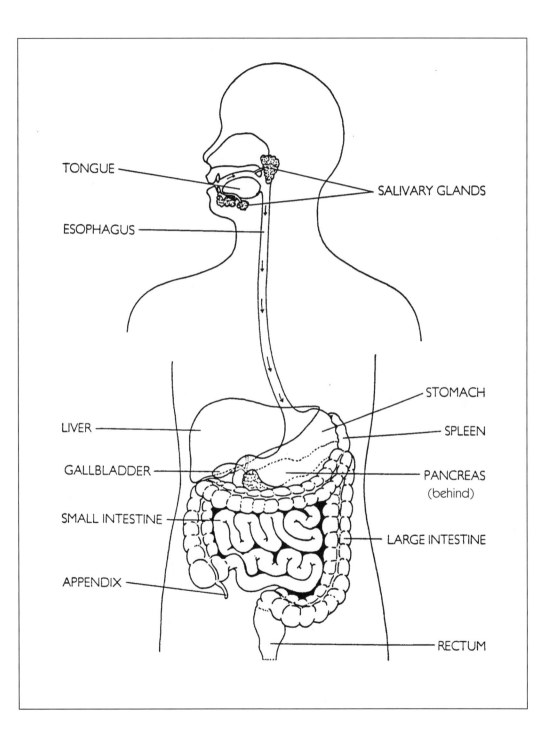

❧ CHLOROPHYLL CLEANSER

Liquid chlorophyll is a famous detoxifier that helps neutralize and deodorize noxious elements in the body's internal mechanisms. It helps oxygenate the entire system and can also be used as an

INGREDIENTS	AMOUNT
liquid chlorophyll	1 T.
pure water (warm)	4 C.

implant. (Implants are explained at the end of this chapter.)

Combine ingredients and fill the enema bag.

❧ BENTONITE CLEANSER

Liquid bentonite is suspended volcanic ash, a special clay hydrated in water by a scientific process, resulting in a product called Sonne's No. 7. Volcanic ash absorbs toxins and aids in the detoxification of

INGREDIENTS	AMOUNT
bentonite (liquid)	1/3 C.
pure water (warm)	4 C.

the alimentary canal. It is a versatile home remedy.

Combine ingredients and fill the enema bag.

Bentonite was first used on a great scale by the British Army in fighting cholera during the Balkan War. Sixty percent of all soldiers who contracted this disease died. When solutions of volcanic ash were introduced, the mortality rate went down to 3 percent. In Europe, the volcanic ash, known as Luvas Healing Earth, "Heilerde," is sold in drug stores; every household carries it in its medicine cabinet. Volcanic ash has one of the world's smallest molecules, shaped like a calling card, which picks up many times its own weight in positive- and negative-charged ions. It is a super detoxifier that assists in absorbing and mobilizing toxins from the bowel wall.

❧ ACIDOPHILUS CLEANSER

Throughout history, humankind has been enjoying the benefits of fermented milk, renowned for its health qualities. It responds wonderfully in the digestive system, promoting the good

INGREDIENTS	AMOUNT
liquid acidophilus or plain yogurt	1/3 C.
pure water (warm)	4 C.

qualities of a healthy colon. Bacterial action in the milk produces a chemical reaction, which digests the milk substances and makes them an ideal food for the human body.

Blend the two together until smooth, then fill the enema bag.

Bacterial action in the large intestine plays a major role in nutrition and digestion. Friendly bacteria also synthesize valuable nutrients by digestion—among others, vitamin K and portions of the B complex vitamins. To a large extent, the flora in the colon determines the state of health in an individual.

Of those influences that greatly alter the bacterial life in the colon, drugs are the most powerful—in particular the "broad spectrum" antibiotics. These drugs can also cause inflammation of the intestinal mucosa. Their chemical reactions are not only hazardous to the well-being of the body; they actually cause disharmony by disrupting the life force.

It takes more than a year, on average, for a new diet to produce any noticeable change in the intestinal flora. A "bridge" food during this time is yogurt. Yogurt has been eaten for centuries in countries from Turkey to Lapland and Iceland to China. It is excellent for keeping healthy bacteria thriving in the intestinal tract; however, all types of yogurt are not equal. They should be sweetened only with spices and fresh fruits. Spices such as cinnamon, nutmeg, and vanilla, added for flavor and digestion, are delicious. Other fermented foods such as sauerkraut, slightly fermented apple juice, Kombucha tea, whey powder, miso, tamari, and kefir milk also foster beneficial bacteria.

The best time to utilize the acidophilus internal bath is after you have completed a fast. This restores the friendly bacteria in your body. The acidophilus acquired its name from the fact that it loves an acid environment. An acid bowel environment is one's best defense against unfriendly bacteria.

Acidophilus is essential after a cleansing fast that is directed to the colon. Acidophilus culture, taken orally in the form of yogurt, in liquid, or in capsules, is helpful in detoxifying the bowel and in building friendly bacteria. It should be continued for at least 30 days orally after completion of any colon-cleansing fast. Acidophilus implants (p. 192) can also be inserted rectally and held overnight. Use ½ cup water and ½ cup acidophilus yogurt or liquid.

❦ COFFEE AND APPLE CIDER VINEGAR CLEANSER

It is helpful when taking coffee enemas to know which type of coffee to choose for each specific ailment. All coffee beans stimulate pineal and pituitary function and are especially good in enemas when cancer has invaded the body. Some coffee beans have digitalis; some stimulate the spleen, others the pancreas. For example, if you are doing a springtime fast for the liver, choose the type of bean that stimulates the liver.[4]

INGREDIENTS	AMOUNT
ground coffee (organic)	2 T.
pure water	2 C.
apple cider vinegar (organic)	2 T.

COFFEE TYPE	ORGAN
Colombian	stomach/heart
Guatemalan	coccyx/pineal
Mexican	pineal
Kenyan	pancreas
New Guinea	spleen
Peruvian	larynx
Salvadoran	tongue
Continental Roast	appendix
Viennese Roast	pituitary
Colombian Supreme	pineal
Jamaican	liver/heart/pineal
Costa Rican	liver
Nicaraguan/Mocha	pineal
Javan	colon
Ethiopian	liver
Indian	spleen

Bring the water to a rolling boil, remove from heat, add the coffee, and let stand for 15 minutes. Add the vinegar. This is enough to mix with about $4^1/_2$ gallons of water.

Strain before using and store unused portion in a cool place. Coffee enemas help bring down the bile from the liver and stimulate the bowel wall to throw out the toxic material faster.

❧ GARLIC CLEANSER

Blend the garlic and water to a smooth liquid, then strain. This amount is enough to mix with about $4^1/_2$ gallons of water. Garlic is a good intestinal cleanser and is particularly

INGREDIENTS	AMOUNT
cloves of garlic, unpeeled (organic)	*4*
pure water	*1 C.*

helpful in ridding the body of parasites. Preventing parasites is always a goal, so do not hesitate to use the Garlic Cleanser any time you like; always use it while undertaking a fast that is directed to a possible parasitic condition.

❧ FLAXSEED CLEANSER

Bring to a boil and let stand for 8 hours or overnight. Strain and discard seeds. Add 4 cups flaxseed tea to 4 to 5 gallons of water used for an enema. Add 1 teaspoon liquid chlorophyll to

INGREDIENTS	AMOUNT
flaxseed	$1/4$ C.
pure water (hot)	6 C.

1 cup flaxseed tea for a cleansing drink. Always use flaxseed tea to help soothe, heal, and lubricate the colon. This formula can be taken orally as a tea as well, 3 times a day.[5] (Flaxseed tea may aid cases of extreme gas, spastic conditions, and ulcerated colitis or serious conditions of colon inflammation.)

❧ SLIPPERY ELM CLEANSER

The herb slippery elm strengthens, heals, and soothes inflamed or irritated areas in the colon, and it absorbs noxious gases.

INGREDIENTS	AMOUNT
pure water	2 C.
slippery elm bark	$1/4$ C.

   Boil the water, turn off heat, add herb. Steep 15 to 20 minutes; strain, cool, and add $1/2$ cup to each quart of pure water to fill your enema bag.

❧ BAYBERRY CLEANSER

The root bark of the bayberry tree contains strong germicidal properties that destroy harmful bacteria in the colon as they tone and cleanse. Hemorrhoids are soothed by the antiseptic qualities of this herb.

INGREDIENTS	AMOUNT
bayberry root bark	2 T.
pure water	2 C.

   Bring ingredients to a boil, cover and simmer for 15 to 20 minutes, cool and strain. Add $1/2$ cup to each quart of pure water to fill your enema bag.

❧ ALOE VERA CLEANSER

Combine the aloe vera with the warm water and use in an enema to help heal the irritated lining of the colon wall. Aloe vera is excellent in controlling unfriendly bacteria in the system.

INGREDIENTS	AMOUNT
aloe vera gel or juice	$1/4$ C.
pure water (warm)	8 C.

It also has anti-inflammatory and antihistamine properties and can be used in various forms to alleviate inflammations throughout the body. Aloe vera is very soothing and healing when used as a colon implant (see below) in the amount of 1/2 cup aloe vera juice or gel and 1/2 cup water. It is important to use aloe vera in a 3-months on and 3-months off pattern for best results. If used over an extended period of time, aloe vera begins to destroy the good bacteria as well as the bad. Therefore, as with all good healing remedies, it should not be overused.

❧ HERBAL CATNIP CLEANSER

One of the best herbal cleansers to use as an enema is catnip tea. Catnip is famous for its sedative effects on the nervous system, and it gently restores the tone of the bowels.

Bring the water to a boil, turn off the heat and add the catnip. Cover and let steep for 30 minutes. Add honey and oils (honey and oils prevent bowel irritation).

INGREDIENTS	AMOUNT
pure water	6 C.
catnip	1/4 C.
honey	1 T.
sesame oil (optional)	2 T.
castor oil (optional)	1 T.

❧ HERBAL COMBINATION CLEANSER

Bring the water to a boil, add the yellow dock or bayberry bark and simmer for 20 minutes. Turn off the heat and add the lobelia leaf or skullcap and steep for 30 minutes, covered tightly. Add the oils and honey. Cool and strain before using.

Lobelia and skullcap are nervines, which help relax the

INGREDIENTS	AMOUNT
pure water	6 C.
yellow dock or bayberry bark or Oregon graperoot	2 heaping T.
lobelia leaf or skullcap	2 heaping T.
sesame oil (optional)	2 T.
castor oil (optional)	1 T.
honey	1 T.

bowel. Yellow dock and bayberry bark are astringents, which help tone the walls of the bowel.

COLON IMPLANTS

All implants are placed in a baby enema syringe and squeezed into the rectum. Combine 1/3 cup distilled water with 1/2 cup acidophilus, aloe vera gel, Flaxseed Tea, or chlorophyll. Insert as much liquid as can be comfortably held. This is best done before bedtime. Expel the contents in the morning.

UPLIFTING BATHS FOR
THE OUTER BODY

❧ BATHS FOR THE OUTER BODY

It is very helpful to take baths during fasting times, since the skin is a major organ of elimination. A bath with steaming water, or a sauna, promotes sweating, which is extremely beneficial in

INGREDIENTS	AMOUNT
fresh-pressed apple juice	2 C.
fresh-pressed celery juice	2 C.
pure water	1 C.

ridding the body of toxins through the skin and lymphatic system. Saunas, mineral or mud baths, aromatic baths, enzyme baths, herbal baths, and body wraps are all excellent companions to aid in the detoxification of the body. It is important to drink plenty of fluids and to avoid feeling overheated. Spend 15 or 20 minutes sweating, then take a cool shower; repeat if desired. While bathing, keep a balance of potassium, calcium, magnesium, and cell salts with this delicious drink.

Blend together and enjoy during your steam bath or treatment. Avoid iced or very cold drinks at all times; they "shock" the body by severely reducing core temperature.

HOME STEAM BATHS

Traditionally, steam baths have been taken in sweat lodges or saunas. American pioneers would wrap a person sitting in a chair in blankets, and place a hot stone in a pail at his or her feet. Then they poured water into the pail so the steam would come up under the blankets, and continued until the person started to perspire.

With modern hot running water and bathtubs, it is not necessary to go to this much trouble. Simply sit in a tub of water as hot as you can tolerate. To the water, add a couple of tablespoons of ginger powder, a handful of rosemary or mint leaves or other aromatic herbs. Put the herbs into a little cloth bag (like a large tea bag) so you do not have to clean them out of the tub. An alternative is to add 1/4 teaspoon of lavender oil, tea tree oil, or some other essential oil. These herbs encourage blood flow to the extremities and stimulate the sweat glands. Drink a fragrant herbal tea or juices before sitting in the bath. To benefit still further from the herbs, mix them with either oatmeal or bran and fill small muslin cotton drawstring bags with this combination. This mixture will make the water soft. Use a good long drawstring so that the bag can hang down, from the hot water tap, deep into the bathtub. The flow of hot water transmits the goodness of the herb as the bath is filled. Eucalyptus and balsam or pine oils, used with sweat baths, hydrotherapy, and massage, are excellent for aiding elimination as well as circulation—preventative as well as healing measures. A good cleansing of the system allows the body forces to function normally in eliminating poisons and congestion.

JAPANESE MISOGI RITUAL

Japanese Shinto religion strongly recommends performing the *misogi* ritual, in which one takes a cold water dip or shower in a river, waterfall, or the ocean. A cold shower after a hot bath of any kind is an excellent way of improving thinking ability and of making the spirit soar.

The best time for this ritual is at midnight or in the early morning. It is necessary to continue for about 10 days in order to have some sign of improvement in thinking. When taking a cold shower, move from the legs up to the front, right shoulder, back, and left shoulder, turning clockwise; then dunk the head last. Anyone who has a weak heart should observe carefully and go easy.

AROMATIC BATHS

Aromatic baths may affect us in a variety of ways. First, there is the fragrance of the essences used—if this is pleasing to the nose, it will also please the spirit. Then there is the physiological action of the essence on the nervous system and the rest of the body,

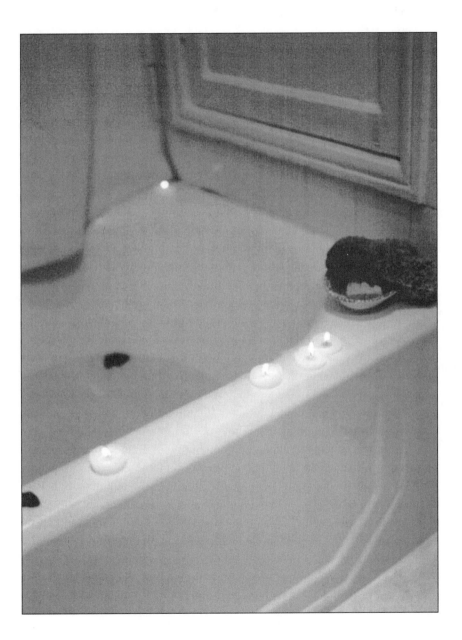

which takes place even though only a very small amount of the oil is absorbed through the skin. A tepid bath (82.5 to 95 degrees) is relaxing and sedative. A hot bath is a tonic if it is short, but it is very debilitating if too long.

ESSENTIAL OILS AND AROMATHERAPY

The use of scented oils played a prominent part in the advanced culture of ancient Egypt. A brilliant man named Imhotep, the king's physician and high priest, is considered the father of aromatherapy.

An ancient Egyptian medical work, the Ebers Papyrus, lists healing formulas, many of which feature aromatic plants. *Kyphi,* perhaps the most famous Egyptian aromatic formula, contained infusions from such herbs as calamus, myrrh, juniper, cinnamon, spikenard, henna, and frankincense. Egyptians burned kyphi at sunset in honor of Ra, the sun god, for its scent as well as for its tranquilizing effect.

According to Eastern philosophers, the vital energy in all living things emanates from what the Chinese call *chi* and the Japanese call *ki.* Every plant manifests this same life force, as do the natural essential oils extracted from them. The subtle energy of these extracts stimulates our own energy fields and establishes a firm basis for healing.

Few people realize that all essential oils are antiseptic. Essential oils stimulate the body's natural defenses by aiding in the formation of phagocytes—white blood cells that consume invading bacteria. In England, essential oils such as lavender and peppermint are used in hospital room vaporizers to cleanse the air, keeping it as germfree as possible to prevent infection. Aromatherapy can relieve symptoms, but primarily aims at the causes of diseases. The main therapeutic action of essential oils is the strengthening of the organs and their functions, while they bolster the defense mechanisms of the body. They do not do the work for the body, but help the body to function bettter. Essences inhibit certain metabolic functions of microorganisms, such as growth and multiplication, eventually destroying them if the action continues.

In France, doctors often prescribe aromatherapy oils for infectious diseases, in place of antibiotics. Other European medical doctors practice aromatherapy extensively, recognizing the healing benefits of aromatic essential oils. These oils protect patients from bacteria, viruses, fungi, parasites, allergens, and toxins.

Since 1887 hundreds of laboratory tests have demonstrated the effectiveness of essential oils as healing agents. For instance, lavender stimulates tissue regeneration after burns, and also soothes sinus infections—as do eucalyptus and peppermint. Peppermint oil is also excellent for relieving headaches and stimulating alertness. When prepared in certain combinations, aromatics have a synergistic effect, making the combinations more effective than the individual oils by themselves. Garlic and hyssop help normalize blood pressure; bergamot and geranium oil stimulate or sedate, depending on the body's particular need. Oil of clove is invaluable for many things, but is especially good for skin cancers, warts, and corns. Clove oil is used in small amounts on the gums for toothache, swollen or sore parts of the mouth, canker sores, insect stings and bites, poison oak, small burns, and sore throat. For those who wish to quit smoking, a small amount on back of the tongue is said to lessen the craving for tobacco. Oil of thyme will destroy fungal infections such as athlete's foot and skin parasites such as scabies, crabs, and lice, when applied externally.

Tea tree oil, prized by the Dreamtime Aborigines, is indigenous to the northern part of Australia's New South Wales. It is a relatively new natural remedy on our continent. The tea tree was so named by a botanist from Captain Cook's expedition in 1770. Some of the crew members had discovered that the leaves of the tree could be brewed into an acceptable tea substitute. There are more than 300 varieties of tea trees, yet only one is known to produce the medicinal oil that has just the right balance of constituents and active ingredients. Terpinen, one active ingredient, must make up 30 percent of the oil to ensure its unique healing properties. Pure tea tree oil is a powerful broad-range antiseptic and bactericide. It is an active antifungal agent and is particularly effective against *Candida albicans* and vaginal infections. Although the oil is very powerful, it has a very low toxicity and is virtually nonirritating. Tea tree oil effectively inhibits throat infections, and pneumonia in laboratory tests. The oil is swabbed directly onto the throat internally. Also a small piece of oil-saturated cloth or cotton is used internally to heal vaginal infections.

Once you begin to use aromatic essential oils, you will wonder how you survived without them. Aromatic oils are excellent to help restore the body during a fast, as well as a delightful therapeutic addition to daily life. The uses for them are many. As with homeopathic remedies, essential oils are more potent in very small doses.

1. Apply essential oils topically at full strength or diluted with vitamin E or castor oil to clean and disinfect cuts, abrasions, insect bites, rashes, and infections.
2. Use rose oil in your bath water, massage oil, skin care lotion, or with an aromatic air diffuser or small inhaler.
3. Add a few drops of rosemary oil to your shampoo or conditioner to treat dandruff or itchy scalp, and thyme oil to your pet's shampoo to help discourage fleas.
4. Gargle with a combination of 3 drops of tea tree oil and 1 cup of hot water to sooth a sore throat; rinse mouth for gum inflammation or toothache pain.

5. Mix 3 drops of tea tree oil with warm water or garlic broth for conditions relating to *Candida albicans*.
6. Mix 5 to 15 drops of tea tree oil in warm water and use as a douche to ease vaginitis.
7. Treat pierced earring wires with essential oils to ward off infections to the ear lobe.
8. Promote clear thinking and alleviate headaches with peppermint oil in an aromatic air diffuser or small inhaler.
9. Clear the sinus cavities by gently inhaling eucalyptus oil in boiling water.
10. Use 7 drops sage oil diluted with biodegradable liquid soap (2 T. in 1 quart water) as a good bug repellent. Put in a spray bottle for use on plants with household bug problems. Plant fresh sage near bug-infested vines, shrubs, trees, and plants.

DRY SKIN BRUSHING

Dry skin brushing is not new. Legend has it that the loofah was discovered when an ancient king offered a great reward to anyone who could find a way to smooth and soften his skin without damaging it. Hence, the use of this natural vegetable sponge. For ages people have used various forms of skin brushing, such as rubbing the skin with coarse plant fibers and loofahs, scrubbing with dry sponges, or brushing the skin with vegetable or boar bristle brushes. In Finland, people vigorously brush their bodies with twigs before entering the sauna. In Turkey, the Turkish towel became famous as a means to rub dead skin off the body before and after the bath. These health practices serve to open the pores and stimulate perspiration.

HOW TO DRY SKIN BRUSH

First acquire an all natural vegetable fiber brush or loofah. Make sure it is not made of synthetic fiber (this can irritate the skin). A long handle is helpful for reaching your back.

Begin by gently brushing with one-stroke movements. The skin should not become red. The basic principle is to brush from the outermost points of your body (hands and feet) toward the center. Start by brushing from your feet to your abdomen, then from your hands up your arms toward your heart. Brush across your upper back and down the front and back of your torso. Cover the entire body surface (except your face) once only.

For your face, use a softer brush since blood vessels are nearer the surface of the skin and can be broken if brushed too hard. Begin in the center of your face and stroke outward. Then brush down the sides of your face and neck. This gentle friction vitalizes your skin and keeps it glowing. The total process takes about 1 to 3 minutes.

Dry skin brushing is a powerful addition to your daily routine, requires only a few minutes, and produces results you can see and feel. My first experience with dry skin brushing was as part of a cleansing fast. I have kept it as part of my schedule to this day. Whether for cleanliness, beauty, or health, the practice of dry skin brushing has continued because it is so beneficial for the body.

Daily dry skin brushing removes the top layer of dead skin with its buildup of dirt and acid, and it deeply cleanses the skin. Unlike soap, which can have a drying effect, skin brushing stimulates the oil-producing glands and assists the body's own moisturizing process. Dry skin brushing is one of the best ways to clean the skin without removing the protective mantle of acid and oils. Most commercial soaps clog the pores and leave a film—much like what is seen if you dip a glass in soapy water, then let it dry. Soap can change the pH balance of the skin, and the chemicals and synthetic perfumes contained in many soaps are absorbed through the pores.

Many health practitioners recommend dry skin brushing as part of a detoxification or internal cleansing program to open up the pores of the skin and clean out the lymphatic system. As the largest organ of elimination, the skin plays a vital role in ridding the body of toxins and impurities that are a potential source of illness. Additionally, brushing increases blood circulation in all underlying organs and tissues.

The best time to dry skin brush is right before your morning shower or bath. Brush the skin when dry, since it may pull and sag if it is brushed wet. Aloe vera is a wonderful skin toner after a dry skin brush massage. It is known as an antibacterial and antifungal. Aloe vera is also well known for soothing burns or sunburns.

ALOE VERA SPRAY

Blend all of the ingredients together. More water may be needed for thinning if aloe vera gel is used. Store the mixture in a small dark-colored glass spray bottle in the refrigerator or a cool place. You will find this especially refreshing for sunburned skin. Pat or rub into skin after a skin brushing.

INGREDIENTS	AMOUNT
aloe vera juice or gel	$^1/_4$ C.
pure water	1 T.
vegetable glycerin	1 tsp.

THYME STEAM BATH

Externally, thyme's antiseptic properties make it a useful mouthwash and a cleansing wash for the skin. It will destroy fungal infections such as athlete's foot and skin parasites. For these purposes, a tincture made from dried thyme and

grain alcohol is used, or the essential oil is applied. The oil is effective when
applied to the joints for rheumatism and sprains.

A bath with thyme is good for nervous disorders. For a bath, soak a bucketful of fresh thyme—or about 2 cups dried thyme—in cold water for 12 hours.
(A smaller quantity is sufficient for children.) Heat the infusion gently after the
soak, and strain it into your bath water. Skin brush. Soak for 20 minutes in the
bath. Keep your heart above water level. Do not dry off when you get out; put
on a robe and get straight into bed. Stay there for an hour so that you work up
a good sweat. Then take a cool shower.[7]

❧ COMFREY STEAM BATH

This plant was known and greatly valued for its medicinal properties in the
Middle Ages. It is extremely useful for diseased and injured bones. Comfrey
baths improve poor circulation in the body in general, and they are good for
itching skin conditions, sore muscles, aches, and pains.

For a bath, soak a bucketful of fresh comfrey or 1 pound of dried comfrey
leaves in cold water for 12 hours, then heat the infusion gently and strain the
liquid into your bathwater. Skin brush. Soak in the bath for 20 minutes, keeping your heart above water level. Do not dry off when you get out; put on a
robe and get straight into bed. Stay there an hour so that you work up a good
sweat. Then take a cool shower.

❧ EPSOM SALTS BATH

This is a good bath for inflamed joints and gout, and for neutralizing and eliminating acids in the system. Epsom salts draws poisons out through the skin and
makes a good skin conditioner bath to relieve itching and sore muscles. Use $1/2$
to 1 cup Epsom salts dissolved in bath water as hot as you can stand it. Keep
your heart above water level. Soak 20 minutes, then take a cool shower.

❧ CALENDULA SITZ BATH

Calendula, or pot marigold, is a member of the aster family. According to an old
folk tradition, the weather can be predicted by watching calendula flowers.
Country folk say that the flowers never open in the morning if rain is on the
way, but if they do open up before 7 A.M., you can be sure of fine weather.

Vaginal fungal infections can be soothed with the help of calendula sitz baths. Soak 1 cup of calendula flowers in 1 gallon of cold water for 12 hours, then heat the infusion gently and strain the liquid into your bathwater. The water should be just deep enough to cover your kidneys. Stay in the bath for 20 minutes. Do not dry off when you get out; put on a robe and get straight into bed. Stay there for an hour so that you work up a good sweat. Then take a cool shower.

❧ YARROW SITZ BATH

Yarrow sitz baths and douches are good treatments for vaginal itching and menopausal symptoms. Follow the same directions used for the calendula sitz bath, using all parts of the yarrow plant.

❧ SULFUR BATHS

One of the most universal remedies to remove lead, arsenic, platinum, gold, and mercury from your body is the sulphur bath. Natural sulphur springs are famous in Europe for healing, and sulfur baths are very popular in many places in the world, not least in North America.

Sulfur is easily overdosed when taken orally, but in a bath the body takes in only what it needs. Once a month, particularly for women following menstruation, a sulphur bath is good to replenish the small amount needed to form the proper amino acid combinations; it also contributes to proper nutrition for the reproductive organs. Sulfur is available in dry form, and the granules or tablets can be added to the bathwater.

Herbs that contain a lot of sulphur are watercress, eyebright, nettle, fennel, mullein, and coltsfoot. These herbs are more effective in supplying natural sulfur when used fresh rather than dried. Soak a bucketful overnight and strain into your bathwater. They may also be eaten raw or brewed into tea.

❧ ROSEMARY AND BENTONITE BATH

This special bath will give results comparable to going to a spa or hot springs for a mud bath and massage, at a fraction of the cost. It is very stimulating, particularly while fasting. Powdered bentonite's unique molecular structure has a negative electrical attraction for positively charged toxins and poisons. Harmful substances are drawn out of the body through a complex interaction of electromagnetic forces and osmosis.

Skin brush. Take 2 or 3 niacin tablets (50 mg each) with fresh-pressed juice, herbal tea, or water. Fill the bathtub with hot water running over a cotton bag filled with 1 cup fresh or ½ cup dried rosemary. Add ½ cup bentonite powdered clay to the water, then 2 or 3 drops of rosemary oil—swish it around to disburse the aroma. Relax in the bath and feel the heat of the niacin flushing your body. After 20 minutes, massage your body thoroughly with a coarse loofah cloth and a little glycerin soap. Add some rosemary oil to your shampoo and finish with a cool shower. This bath is a treat. You will feel great and smell wonderful.

✿ EUCALYPTUS AND PINE BATHS

The simple addition of eucalyptus oil to bathwater is very effective for colds, bronchial problems, hay fever, and asthma. Do not add the oil until you are in the water, then begin by slowly adding from 3 to 6 drops at a time. Swish the water around to disburse the scent. Then add more after 10 minutes. End the bath with a cool shower.

The leaves of eucalyptus branches, such as those found in flower shops, are an excellent decongestant when boiled and the steam is gently inhaled. Pine needles and pine oil are also very soothing for all bronchial difficulties.

✿ SEA WATER BATH

The seas are rich in minerals that are absorbed through the skin, and help nourish the glands. If you can go to the seashore, do so as regularly as possible. As a substitute, the following bath is as close to the real thing as possible.

INGREDIENTS	AMOUNT
Epsom salts	1 C.
sea salt	1 C.

Dissolve the salts in a tub of tepid water (not too warm) and soak for up to 30 minutes. Lightly shower afterward without using too much soap.

❧ SEA SALT BATH

This bath is excellent to take particularly after receiving X-ray treatments, to diminish the effects of radiation.

Skin brush first. To your bathwater, add 4 to 5 pounds of sea salt, stirring to dissolve. While soaking in the bath, sip 1 or 2 cups of miso broth. Stay in the bath for 20 to 30 minutes, then finish with a cool shower.

❧ THE BAVARIAN OIL BATH

The famed healer Father Sebastian Kneipp used this bath at his healing clinic in Bavaria. He put his patients on an all-natural diet, and emphasized bathing as a means of helping to boost sluggish glands and sleepy hormones to promote overall mental and physical health.

INGREDIENTS	AMOUNT
corn or olive oil	1/4 C.
rose geranium oil	1 tsp.
liquid soap or shampoo	1 T.

Stir oils and soap into a tub of comfortably warm water. Soak for up to 30 minutes, then finish with a cool shower.

❧ MEDITERRANEAN OIL BATH

A handful of any cold-pressed seed oil (olive, wheat germ, peanut, corn, sunflower) in a tub of water is soothingly relaxing to your glands and skin. Soak for about 30 minutes. Then to rid your skin of dead cells, combine 1/2 cup sugar with enough oil to dampen the mixture. Massage this exfoliating scrub all over your body and face before you shower with a light soaping and rinse. Repeat once or twice a month to improve your skin clarity and softness and stimulate your glandular system.

❧ BUFFALO BIRD WOMAN BATH

This special bath was created to honor Buffalo Bird Woman, a Native American who was known for her talent in building round houses.

INGREDIENTS	AMOUNT
jojoba oil	1 tsp.
sage oil	4 to 6 drops

Stir oils into a tub of comfortably warm water. Soak for up to 30 minutes, then finish with a cool shower.

🌿 FRESH FLOWER BATHS

Any bath with fresh flowers floating in it is very healing, especially during times of emotional difficulty and trauma. Go into your garden and pick a bowl of fragrant fresh blossoms. Add them to your bath after you have settled into the water. Close your eyes and sprinkle them around, or have a friend help you. When you open your eyes, you will be delighted! (Be sure to strain the flowers from your bathwater before draining.)

🌿 MAID MARIAN'S BEAUTIFYING BATH

Gather 2 handfuls of oak leaves and 1 handful of the leaves of an elder tree on a fine spring morning (9–10 A.M.). Put them in your bath with a drop of lavender oil, and you will rise from it refreshed, serene, and beautiful.[8]

🌿 DR. JARVIS'S APPLE CIDER VINEGAR BATH

Some soaps upset the pH balance of your skin, and overuse can cause the skin and scalp to itch. Instead of using soap, add $1/2$ cup apple cider vinegar to your bath water, and remain for 15 minutes. Use as little soap as possible, and apply a mild solution of cider vinegar and water to keep the acid mantle in your skin balanced.[9]

Important Note: To protect the quality of our water supplies and to care for our skins, always use biodegradable soaps.

MASSAGE THERAPY

Take not just a few minutes, but set a period and make of it an occasion when the massage is given. Take from 30 minutes to an hour, or hour and a half to do it! [1688-7]

For the cleaning of the system allows the body-forces themselves to function normally, and thus eliminate poisons, congestions, and conditions that would become acute through the body.[10] [257-254]

—Edgar Cayce

MASSAGE AND MANIPULATION

Manipulation and massage therapy rank among the oldest and most instinctive of all the healing methods. One naturally reacts, when hurt or in pain, by stroking or rubbing the affected areas; a mother soothes a crying baby by stroking its head or back. Psychologists confirm that this stroking is not only soothing to the baby, but plays an important role in its mental and emotional development. Animals lick their wounds to cleanse and hasten healing by increasing the flow of blood to the area. They rub themselves against the bark of a tree or other rough surfaces to massage their heads, sides, and backs, sometimes to cleanse or heal—other times for the sheer delight of it. All animal trainers use some method of stroking in their work.

There are written records of massage being utilized as far back as 3000 B.C. by the Chinese and forward through history by the Japanese, Burmese, Hindus, Persians, Russians, Egyptians, Polynesians, Greeks, Romans, Italians, the Swedes, and the French. In the first century B.C., the learned Roman physician Galen advocated manipulation in the treatment of disease and in the general maintenance of health.

Swedish massage practitioners have finally overcome the "bad press" in our country, as massage is becoming more accepted. The nineteenth century Swedish physiologist, poet, fencing master, and founder of the Swedish massage system, Peter Henrik Ling, brought the knowledge and some of the practices of the ancients up to date. Much of the improved technique in manipulation and medical gymnastics has stemmed from Ling's efforts to methodize this field on a scientific basis. In 1874 Dr. Andrew Taylor Still introduced osteopathic medicine into the healing arts and, twenty years later, Daniel David Palmer founded chiropractic.

The two world wars greatly upgraded the science of rehabilitation in the treatment of veterans. Although for many years the medical profession was reluctant to use the full therapeutic range of massage and manipulation, war conditions impelled the medical establishment to accept the healing role of massage and manipulation in physical medicine.

Manipulation is basically massage therapy that is usually given with the hands. The techniques vary with people and place; sometimes the feet, elbows, or forearms are also used. Massage can be both stimulating and relaxing. Quiet stroking of the body brings about a relaxing semi-hypnotic feeling that has a more favorable effect on the nervous system than tranquilizers or sleeping pills, with none of the side effects. Pressure and stretching are also used, along with active and passive movements of the joints, muscles, connective tissue, tendons, and ligaments.

Massage affects every part of the body—nerves, organs, glands, circulation, and muscle tone—helping to rid the body of toxins and fatigue poisons. When massage is administered by someone with a healing attitude and ability, enzyme activity as well as circulation can be influenced. Awareness and attunement are important keys in healing, particularly in massage therapy.

The skin plays an important role in assimilation and elimination. Therefore, special attention to lubricants used on the skin is important because they effect specific results for each individual. The following massage mixtures can be used to achieve specific results depending on the needs of the individual receiving the massage. Prepare them yourself and ask your massage therapist to use the preparation on you during treatment, or use the oils for self-massage.

❧ BASIC COMPLEXION OIL

For use as a basic massage oil. Shake well before use.

INGREDIENTS	AMOUNT
organic peanut oil	$^3/_4$ C.
virgin olive oil	$^1/_4$ C.
rose water	$^1/_4$ C.
vegetable glycerin	1 T.

❧ PEANUT AND OLIVE OIL

This recipe is recommended for those who suffer from arthritis, rheumatism, Parkinson's disease, multiple sclerosis, the aftereffects of anesthesia, kidney disorders, toxemia, injuries from accidents, and menopausal complaints.

INGREDIENTS	AMOUNT
peanut oil	¼ C.
olive oil	¼ C.
lanolin (liquefied)	1 tsp.

Peanut or olive oil alone is very good to use for paralysis, apoplexy, palsy, polio, low vitality, fatigue, poor circulation, coronary occlusion, ulcerated stomach, and glandular disturbance.

❧ CASTOR OIL

Castor oil is recommended for arthritis, back pain, muscle and joint pain, contractions, and spasms. Warm the oil slightly for better penetration into the skin and add a few drops of rose oil if you prefer. Use a mixture of 1 teaspoon castor oil, 3 drops of vitamin E oil, and 2 drops tea tree oil as a treatment for keeping the vaginal walls healthy and infection-free. Massaging this inner area with the oil can be helpful for women of all ages.

❧ MYRRH OIL

Myrrh oil is especially good for the lower limbs, varicose veins, tendinitis, strains, and fractures.

Heat, but do not boil, equal amounts of olive oil and tincture of myrrh to massage into knees, limbs, and feet, right after these have been bathed in hot water. Or, make an ointment by first gently heating powdered myrrh until it becomes aromatic. Remove from heat and add an equal amount of olive oil. If the knee or kneecap is injured, use plain salt dissolved in pure apple cider vinegar the day after injury as a massage rub to supply calcium, acids, and oils that will prevent accumulation of water. Alternate between this formula and the myrrh oil for up to 1 month.

BONESET AND CATNIP TEA FOR MASSAGE, BROKEN BONES, AGING, AND ENERGY

Some professional movement and massage therapists wisely offer this tea 1 hour before massage to produce the heightened effects of massage and more responsiveness from the body. It relaxes sore muscles, even strained muscles, with phenomenal results. Make the tea yourself and drink it before a scheduled appointment for massage.

❧ BONESET AND CATNIP TEA FOR MASSAGE

The effects of the boneset teas depend largely on how they are taken and the preparation and strength of the teas.

Steep herbs in boiled water for 20 minutes, or more if desired. Strain.

INGREDIENTS	AMOUNT
dried catnip	3 T.
dried boneset	3 T.
pure water	4 C.

Boneset is a plant that has tremendous healing and rejuvenating properties. It is used as a healing herb to mend broken bones in half the time normally needed, and is effective for the pain, swollen joints, and stiffness. A cup of boneset tea a day is good for arthritis or rheumatism. It is considered a tonic against aging, or for keeping energy up, colds away, and the body moving freely. Drink boneset tea at the first sign of fever or sniffles, for quick relief.

CHAPTER EIGHT

HERBS

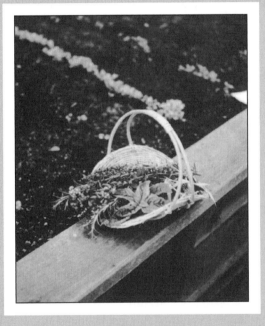

PLANTS WISH US WELL IN EVERY WAY. THEY CAN
PROVIDE NOT ONLY FOR OUR PHYSICAL NEEDS, BUT
ALSO FOR OUR HEART AND SOUL. THEY ARE PER-
FECTLY WILLING TO BRING US THE BLESSINGS OF
THEIR UNION WITH NATURE. BUT, AS THE PLAN-
TAIN SPIRIT TOLD ME, THEY CAN DO NOTHING
UNLESS THEY ARE ASKED.[1]

—ELIOT COWAN

HERBS

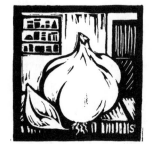

Long before records were kept, humankind was using wild herbs for food and medicine. In early biblical times, the Hebrews used herbs as healthy flavorsome foods. Many of the culinary herbs of today are native to the Middle East. The thymes, sages, mints, and marjorams grew in the Bible lands as did rosemary and hyssop; coriander and cumin came from Egypt. About 2000 B.C. in Babylon, we find the first documented account of herbal remedies. It described tried and tested medicinal uses of herbs, and included many herbs that are well-known today, such as bay tree, thyme, caraway, and coriander.

The ancient Egyptians imported many of their herbs, spices, and aromatic oils from Babylon and from distant India, learning the many traditional uses for these substances from their traders. Anise, caraway, fenugreek, opium, thyme, saffron, and others were in great demand for foods, medicines, cosmetics, dyes, perfumes, and disinfectants.

In their turn, the ancient Greeks built upon earlier knowledge of herbs, adding greatly to it. Most important were the medical writings of Hippocrates, the "Father of Medicine," who was a physician and teacher. About 400 B.C., his students were being taught the value of herbs in easing pain and curing disease.

The Romans had a vast knowledge of herbs. Such was their faith in the ability of herbs to heal sickness and maintain good health that, as they conquered most of Europe, they carried herb seeds and plants wherever they went to cultivate and use. Over 200 different herbs were introduced to Britain by the invading Romans; among them were fennel, sage, borage, betony, parsley, rosemary, and thyme. During the 400 years of Roman occupation, many of the herbs they cultivated so carefully became naturalized and now grow wild.

In 1597 Gerard, an apothecary to James I, produced his well-known *Herbal*. It was based on the work of the Flemish physician Dodoens, but it included many of the plants growing in America, "that new lande." He mentioned the potato and the tomato, which he called "Apple of Love," as well as those herbs growing in his own physic garden.[2]

Among their few belongings, those first settlers in the Americas brought with them the treasured seeds and roots of their favorite herbs. Many quickly flourished in their new environment, while Native Americans showed the new inhabitants which indigenous plants had culinary and medicinal value. The best known of these was bergamot, the leaves of which the Native Americans used as a tea; for them the gateway to the spirit world was through medicinal plants and their healing properties.

The cultivation of herbs in North America reached its peak in the eighteenth century with the emergence of the Shakers—so-called because of their religious dances. The Shaker economy was based on agriculture; they became our professional herbalists, the first to grow and sell medicinal herbs on a large scale. The influence of the Shakers lasted for more than 100 years and, as a result, the interest in herbs continued in this country without interruption. In Britain, however, the custom of growing herbs for use in the home had largely died out by the mid-nineteenth century because of the Industrial Revolution and the rise of an urban society. Small, terraced lots for houses in the quickly growing towns offered no space for gardens. In less heavily industrialized countries such as France and Italy, the use of herbs, particularly in cooking, has never ceased.

During the twentieth century, advances in scientific knowledge have enabled scientists to isolate the chemical substances of plants and to synthesize their properties. This meant that accurate doses of a drug could be administered and "instant" medicine from the drug-store became available to all. And synthetic herbal flavorings sold in little bottles were simple to use in the kitchen.

During the past thirty-five years, there has been a dramatic revival of interest in herbs on both sides of the Atlantic. Bulk processing and the addition of preservatives to food has resulted in loss of natural flavor, color, and aroma. The palate is dulled by these artificial agents, and many people are anxious to use herbs again in order to taste their delicious natural flavoring and to benefit from their nutritional qualities. The value and pleasure that herbs have to offer are, happily, once more being recognized.

The use of herbs can be a very simple healing art. They are invaluable nutritional supplements for restoring and rebuilding the body internally—in the form of teas, tinctures, powders as herbal wines, in gelatin capsules and pills, and added to vegetable or fruit juices and foods. Herbs are even smoked for lung and throat upsets and are a very pleasant substitute for tobacco, imparting a lovely aroma and taste to the palate. Externally, herbs are utilized to great effect in baths, oils, ointments, salves, poultices, plasters, and liniments. They should be incorporated into daily life to build the body and to strengthen the mind and spirit. Locally grown herbs should be used for the same reason that local fruits, vegetables, and other foods are preferred—they contain hundreds of local bio-chemical constituents that may have a better effect on the body. Just as the climate and outward conditions of our lives affect our characteristics and personality, so also do the growing conditions of a specific area affect the characteristics of foods that can be found growing there.

Herbs are very important to use while fasting because of their detoxifying, eliminating, building, and sustaining qualities. Herbs help maintain and stabilize the body through a fasting and cleansing diet and help to stave off hunger pangs. Many different herbs can have curative effects on the same illness or disease; however, there are usually a specific few that have a greater effect because of their chemical makeup. These are the ones that ultimately become the most well-known treatments or remedies.

HERBAL ESSENTIALS

In cases of advanced illness, using *fresh* herbs daily may be the best way of achieving a complete recovery. When the ailment is not so serious, *dried* herbs may be given. If you gather them from the wilderness, you must know your herbs very well so as not to make a mistake. Learning from books is not always the best way; befriend an expert and ask to be instructed. In most areas, fresh herbs can be gathered from the earliest stirrings of spring until the end of November, and there are some, such as rosemary, that can be gathered year-round. Roots are best extracted in the early spring or fall; leaves should be gathered before and during the time of flowering. When it is the flowers you need, take them just as the herb flowering season begins. Fruits should be collected as they are beginning to ripen fully. It is best to gather herbs in the morning when the dew is gone, or at noon, when the volatile oils are most active.

Pick the herbs from strong healthy plants, taking care to avoid hurting the plant so that it will continue to grow vigorously. Place the herbs in a wide, flat basket while gathering them. Before preparing them, sprinkle or spray the herbs with water and shake dry, or better still, if you know your gathering spot is clean, do not wash them at all. All roots and barks have to be washed well before drying. Herbs must be dried quickly in a warm, airy, shaded room. Test your herbs for dryness; if they are brittle and snap, then the job is done. Put them in green glass jars to protect them from sunlight or, if you have only plain glass, put them in a cupboard. Do not keep them forever. When spring comes again, clear them out and gather a fresh harvest. They lose their properties over time. When the herbs have served their purpose, put them in the compost heap to enrich the soil.

There are 3 methods of brewing tea, depending on the types of plants used, personal preference, and the end result desired. These methods are infusion, solar/lunar, and decoction.

INFUSION

Fresh herbs are first bruised by rubbing between the hands or using a mortar and pestle to break up the tissue structure and release the active principles. If fresh herbs are to be used, the amount is doubled because much of the weight of the fresh herb is water. To utilize the volatile oils in herbs such as the mints or eucalyptus, or the delicate plant parts such as flowers and soft leaves, the herbs are steeped in a tightly covered container or pot.

❧ STANDARD MEDICINAL HERBAL TEA

Bring the water to a boil in a glass or stainless-steel pot with a lid, and pour it over the herbs. Steep in a tightly covered vessel, allowing from 10 to 30 minutes. This method is called an infusion. The herbs are not boiled because that destroys their medicinal qualities.

INGREDIENTS	AMOUNT
pure water	2 C.
dried herb (double amount if fresh)	3 T.

SOLAR/LUNAR TEA

A solar tea or lunar tea is made by exposing the herbs in a tightly covered glass bottle or jar of water to the sun or moon for 1 or 2 days or nights. This is a fun method for children. Aromatic leaf herbs or flowers work best—peppermint, hibiscus flowers, lemongrass, red clover flowers, rosemary, orange or lemon peel, chamomile flowers, or any green herbs. Herbal teas are delicious when combined equally with fresh organic apple juice; this combination is pleasing to children and adults alike, served as a warm or cool drink. The variations can be endless. Using herbal drink combinations in place of less desirable beverages—such as sodas, alcohol, coffee, milk, and canned juices—will both fortify the body with superior nutrition and aid in its constant restorative processes.

DECOCTION

To extract the deeper essences from coarser leaves, stems, barks, and roots, the herbs are simmered for 30 to 60 minutes. This method is called a decoction. In many cases, the herbs are simmered uncovered and the volume of water is decreased by half through evaporation. However, some of these coarser herbs, such as burdock root, cinnamon, and valerian, contain important volatile oils. These must be gently simmered or steeped in a covered pot.

COMBINING DECOCTION AND INFUSION

Occasionally, a formula will combine roots and bark with soft leaves and flowers. To make such a tea, a decoction is first made with the coarser materials; then it is strained and poured over the delicate plant parts. This is steeped, tightly covered, for 10 to 30 minutes.

Medicinal infusions and decoctions are very strong, not like the weak beverage teas familiar to most people. The standard daily amount to use is $\frac{1}{2}$ to 1 cup taken 3 times daily. Frequent small amounts of 2 to 3 tablespoons taken every 30 minutes are also effective.

Any medicinal tea may be made weaker by adding more water or diluting it in fruit or vegetable juice. For convenience, prepare at one time enough tea for 3 days and keep it refrigerated in a tightly closed jar. Herb teas generally will not keep more than 3 days this way. They should be gently reheated (not boiled) in a covered pot when needed, or served as a cool, blended drink.

HERBAL MINERAL FORMULA

This delicious herbal syrup supplies easily assimilated minerals such as iron, calcium, silicon, magnesium, potassium, sulfur, iodine, zinc, and trace minerals. It is good for all deficient and anemic conditions. If you enjoy the taste of molasses, this beverage is a pleasant addition to your daily diet, and it is useful in many restorative cleansing fasts. The rich syrup may be enjoyed by the tablespoonful once or twice a day or used to sweeten herbal teas and fruit or vegetable juices. The herbs used may be fresh or dry, but double the amount if fresh herbs are used.

❧ RECIPE

Simmer root herbs slowly, uncovered, in a glass or stainless-steel saucepan until the volume of water is reduced by half. Strain the liquid into a bowl; return the herbs to the saucepan and add enough water to just cover them. Simmer for 10 minutes more. Strain and combine the two liquids, and again simmer until reduced by half. Pour over leaf herbs. Cover tightly and allow to steep for 20 to 30 minutes. Strain and measure the liquid, then add an equal amount of blackstrap molasses. Store in a tightly covered glass jar in a cool place or refrigerate. Enjoy 1 tablespoon 2 to 4 times daily, where flexibility is allowed during a fast. This syrup is also good to take any time for any deficient conditions.

INGREDIENTS	AMOUNT
pure water	4 C.
comfrey root	1 T.
parsley root	1 T.
yellow dock root	1 T.
horsetail	1 T.
kelp	1 T.

INGREDIENTS	AMOUNT
parsley leaf	1 T.
nettles	1 T.
Irish moss	1 T.
watercress	1 T.
blackstrap molasses	as called for

❧ ANISE AND FENNEL TEA

The seeds of anise and fennel contain sources of plant estrogen that can act as natural estrogen for women, helping to ease the emotional swings and hot flashes associated with menopause.

INGREDIENTS	AMOUNT
fennel seed	1½ T.
pure water	2 C.
anise seed	1½ T.

Boil the fennel seeds in water for 15 to 20 minutes; add the anise seeds, cover and steep 15 minutes. Cool, strain, and drink as a tea or add to juices for variation.

❧ SEXY SARSAPARILLA TEA

The herb sarsaparilla is one of the most important natural hormone rejuvenators. It contains both testosterone, the male sex hormone, and progesterone, the female sex hormone. This herb is valued for treating venereal diseases, sexual impotence, menopausal problems, and to balance hormones in men and women.

INGREDIENTS	AMOUNT
sarsaparilla root	2 T.
false unicorn or black cohosh root	2 T.
pure water	3 C.
fresh lemon rind or juice (organic)	optional

Sarsaparilla is high in iron and other minerals and vitamins that also make it effective as a blood purifier, and for rheumatism and skin diseases—by stimulating the body's defense system.

Bring the roots and water to a boil, cover, and simmer for 15 to 20 minutes. Cool and strain. Add lemon if desired. Drink ½ cup before meals. This can be combined with fresh juices for variety.

❧ GINGER TEA

Wild ginger is a native North American plant whose medicinal qualities were known to many Indian tribes. It is one of the most versatile herbal stimulants. Gingerroot tea is of great benefit to the stomach, lungs, intestines, kidneys, bladder, and

INGREDIENTS	AMOUNT
fresh gingerroot (sliced)	3 to 5 inch piece
pure water	4 to 5 C.
maple syrup	4 T.
lemon juice	1 lemon

uterus by equalizing circulation. Try this favorite recipe for gingerroot tea. It is delicious. I like to serve this instead of coffee after dinner to promote digestion. Guests love it!

Simmer the root in water for 30 minutes. Cool the tea. Add maple syrup and lemon juice. Dried gingerroot can also be used in the proportion of 1 teaspoon per cup of water.

❧ FRESH TURMERIC GINGER TEA

This tea is excellent for fasting 1 or 2 days, or as an addition to a juice fast. It is a very good substitute for coffee, as ginger can be quite stimulating.

Note: If fresh turmeric root is unavailable, make the tea with only the ginger and licorice root.

Simmer roots in water for 20 to 30 minutes, cool slightly. Add syrup and lemon juice. This tea is delicious warm or chilled.

INGREDIENTS	AMOUNT
fresh turmeric root (sliced)	*2-inch piece*
fresh gingerroot (sliced)	*2-inch piece*
dried licorice root (optional)	*4-inch portion*
pure water	*6 C.*
maple syrup	*¹⁄₄ C.*
lemon	*to taste*

❧ "CHOCOLATE" PEPPERMINT TEA

This tea has a nicely balanced rich flavor of "chocolate" peppermint, but with minerals and vitamins galore. Kuchica twig tea is higher in calcium than milk.

Boil the kuchica twig in water for 10 minutes and remove from heat. Add the remaining herbs, cover tightly, and steep for 20 to 30 minutes. Strain before drinking.

INGREDIENTS	AMOUNT
kuchica twig	*¹⁄₄ C.*
peppermint leaves	*2 T.*
red clover leaves	*2 T.*
red raspberry leaves	*2 T.*
yarrow	*1 T.*
pure water	*6 C.*

❧ PEPPERMINT TEA

Peppermint, a great herb for year-round use, has always been a common household remedy, and grows prolifically in most any garden. Drinking peppermint leaf tea during fasting and cleansing freshens the breath and body odor, and it is stimulating as well. Peppermint is a standard infusion tea. Inhaled as an aromatic oil, it is excellent to relieve headache and sinus pressure. It is also a nice cooling herb—iced peppermint tea is a good balance during hot summer weather.

INGREDIENTS	AMOUNT
pure water	4 C.
peppermint leaves	1 T.
elder flowers	1 T.

Use the standard recipe for a peppermint leaf tea or try this combination for colds and fevers.

Bring water to a boil in a glass or stainless steel saucepan. Remove from heat and add the herbs. Allow to steep for 15 to 20 minutes. Drink up to 3 cups per day for adults and 1 to 2 cups for children. Get under lots of blankets with a hot water bottle. Sweating should begin in 30 minutes and continue through the night to help relieve a fever or cold.

PAU D'ARCO BEAUTIFUL SKIN TEA

Pau d'arco is an herb that benefits the whole body. It kills viruses and fungi as it builds the immune system. Tasty too!

INGREDIENTS	AMOUNT
pure water	4 C.
whole cloves	1½ T.
peppermint	2 T.
pau d'arco bark	4 T.

Combine water and cloves, bring to a boil and simmer 10 minutes. Turn off heat. Add peppermint and pau d'arco bark, cover, steep 15 minutes and strain.

THYME TEA

In some parts of Europe, thyme is considered a holy plant, dedicated to the Virgin Mary, and in Austria wreaths and garlands of thyme are still taken to church to be blessed on

INGREDIENTS	AMOUNT
dried thyme (double if fresh)	3 T.
pure water	2 C.

the festival of Corpus Christi. Thyme can be used in an unusually wide variety of ways. It is important as a parasiticide for intestinal worms, for bronchial problems, cough, laryngitis, shortness of breath, and to clear the system of impurities. Thyme tea combinations are delicious when sweetened with ½ teaspoon maple or brown rice syrup.

Boil, then steep for 20 minutes and strain. Combine equal parts of these herbs for variety:

- thyme, lavender, comfrey
- thyme, mullein, red clover
- thyme, rosemary, sage
- thyme, comfrey, anise

Drinking a cup of thyme tea in the morning instead of black coffee or tea can really work wonders. Your stomach will be very grateful to you, and you will find that you feel fresher and more wide-awake and full of get-up-and-go. If you have a tendency to start the day with coughing fits, thyme tea is useful.

🌿 GET-THE-LEAD-OUT TEA

It is important to cleanse the system of lead residue. Lead is a protoplasmic poison—it interferes with the life energy–enzyme exchange in the living body. Only people living in very isolated areas are free from lead ingestion; it is either in the foods we eat or in the air we breathe. This is a wonderful herbal formula for removing lead from the body.

INGREDIENTS	AMOUNT
pure water	4 C.
basil	1 T.
rosemary	1 T.
hyssop	1 T.
boneset	1 T.

In a glass or stainless steel pan, boil the water. Remove from heat and add the herbs. Cover tightly and allow to steep for 20 minutes. Strain and drink 1 cup 3 times daily.

🌿 CINNAMON ORANGE TEA

An excellent tea can be made with fresh or dried organic orange peel and cinnamon stick. This tea is refreshing served warm or cold, any time of year, to stimulate the liver and gallbladder and to purify the blood and body in general.

INGREDIENTS	AMOUNT
pure water	4 C.
fresh orange peel (organic)	1/2 C.
cinnamon stick	1

Boil the water; add fresh or dried orange peel in the quantity of 1 or 2 oranges according to taste, along with the cinnamon stick. Cover tightly and simmer for 30 minutes. Allow to cool. Enjoy warm or cool.

KOMBUCHA (TEA CIDER)

Kombucha tea has been highly valued in Asia and Europe for hundreds of years as a natural remedy, and for good reason. The range of medicinal uses for this tea extends from the slightest indisposition to the gravest illness.

Russian research, in particular, has shown that many of the substances in kombucha tea have antibiotic and detoxicating properties. They also play a vital role in the biochemical processes in the human body. In contrast to many drugs, with their unpleasant side effects, the active substances in Kombucha work on the system as a whole. They are beneficial to the metabolism and can restore the cell membranes to normal without side effects, thus promoting general health and well-being.[3]

Knowledge of and use of the Kombucha culture was forgotten during the Second World War, but it is being reintroduced. Many naturopaths prescribe the delicious Kombucha tea for their patients to stimulate the whole glandular system, to improve immunity and metabolism, for constipation, also for hemorrhoids, arteriosclerosis, high blood pressure, gout, rheumatism, headaches, diabetes, tonsillitis, dysentery, anxiety, irritability, and skin rashes on the face. Our elders remember it as sponge tea.[4]

The preparation of Kombucha tea begins with obtaining the self-renewing culture of the Kombucha tea fungus; this cohesive mixture of organisms transforms simple sweetened tea into a lightly sweet, slightly sparkling, cool amber beverage that tastes like fruity wine. One Kombucha culture can be maintained for a lifetime; in past times, it was passed down in families as a healing agent. Kombucha has been used as a detoxifying beverage in clinical work and for prevention of disease in the home. Glucuronic acid, a key detoxifier abundant in Kombucha, aids the liver in processing excessive amounts of freely circulating toxic substances. It is, therefore, an excellent detoxifier and body builder while a person is fasting, as well as in the general diet. Refer to Sources for mail order.[5]

Note: The formation of alcohol in Kombucha tea depends largely on the constituent yeasts in the culture, the fermentation temperature, and the amount of sugar used. A normal homemade preparation should probably reach an average alcohol content of around 0.5 percent, or slightly higher. This is the amount present in so-called alcohol-free beer, many fruit juices, and some types of white bread. Rehabilitated alcoholics should refrain from the use of Kombucha and alcohol-free beer.

CHAPTER NINE

WISDOM CHARTS

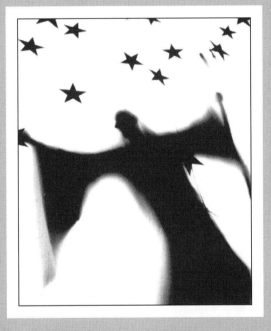

STUDY THOSE CHARTS PERTAINING TO
KEEPING WELL BALANCED IN THE CHEMI-
CAL FORCES OF THE BODY. NOT IN SUCH
A WAY AS TO BECOME A HUMAN PILLBOX,
BUT RATHER TO KNOW THE LAW AND TO
KEEP IT. [1] [2981-3]

—EDGAR CAYCE

THE BALANCING ACT

"Diet is an extremely important factor in creating balance needed for even distribution of energy in physical, mental and spiritual activities. One should begin by obeying the laws of balanced eating. A deliberate choice of food that is known to be harmful, or the refusal to choose food believed to be good, builds blocks at the subconscious level, preventing a person from recognizing the guidance which is continually available to him or her. Real guidance for choices can come from the unconscious as an individual takes a step along the path he or she believes to be right. The process of bringing oneself to these small first steps in self-discipline is far more important than blind choice of some new fad diet." [2]

ACID AND ALKALINE

Many people are completely unaware of the importance of applying the proper balance of food types in the daily diet. For optimal energy and to maintain health, a balance between the acids and the alkalis of the body is essential. The acid-alkaline balance varies with the individual and his or her stress level. Generally it ranges between 75 percent and 85 percent alkaline-producing foods to between 15 percent and 25 percent acid-producing foods in the diet.

In humans, organs such as the kidneys and the large intestine eliminate waste and toxins, maintaining the internal environment in the most ideal condition. However, there are limitations: If we eat too many poison-producing foods, or not enough of the materials needed to clean out poisons, then our internal environment changes beyond the body's control. It deviates from the optimum conditions in which our cells can live, and the cells become sick and die. Many illnesses are the result of the body's attempt to clean up its internal environment. The body secretes and maintains many different kinds of fluids; the most important is blood, which has a pH level of 7.4—slightly alkaline. This alkalinity has to be kept almost constant; even minor variations are dangerous. With too acid blood, the heart relaxes and ceases to beat; with too alkaline blood, it contracts and ceases to beat.

The most striking observation one can make about the general North American diet is how overabundant the acid-producing foods are in the daily food intake of most individuals. This problem is intensified while traveling because most restaurants do not offer high-quality vegetable, fruit, and grain dishes to balance out the concentrated protein foods such as meat, fish, and poultry.

Our bodies have built-in regulators—called blood buffers—to prevent increased acidity that work to keep the pH from fluctuating. For instance, exercise and movement make the blood more acid, but breathing deeply and rapidly for a minute or two is the body's natural way of decreasing this acidity.

An individual with too much acid in the system will experience all manner of adverse physical dysfunctions, such as a susceptibility to colds and flus. Conversely, an individual who maintains a system that is mostly alkaline will experience good general health and well-being. This is not to say that alkaline is better than acid in the system, but that the amount of acidity needed to maintain health is far less than the amount of alkaline chemical action. The balance of the two is essential.

When ingested, all foods are either acid- or alkaline-producers. All natural foods contain both acid- and alkaline-forming elements; in some, acid-forming elements dominate, in others, it is the reverse. It is not the organic matter of foods that leaves acid or alkaline residues in the body, but the inorganic matter (sulphur, phosphorus, potassium, sodium, magnesium, and calcium) that determines the acidity or alkalinity of the body fluids.

Foods comparatively rich in acid-forming elements are generally high protein—animal products and most grains. Foods comparatively rich in alkaline-forming elements are most fruits and vegetables. Alkaline grains are millet, buckwheat, and sprouted grains.

The most common causes of an overly acidic condition are the over-consumption of fats, proteins, sugars, white flour products, and milled white rice. Chemicals added to or absorbed by foods—such as coloring, preservatives, pesticides, and synthetic drugs—are also acid to the system. Another dangerous combination is sugar and animal foods eaten together. Taken separately, protein and sugar are not so harmful; Eskimos consume a lot of animal foods but not much sugar, and they have a low incidence of cancer. Primitive Eskimos, who consume as much as ten pounds of meat daily—consisting of raw fish and blubber—have hardly any signs of circulatory diseases. The reason they do not develop vascular diseases is because most of the food they consume is raw. The body does not have to secrete large amounts of enzymes, because the food is in an easily digestible state. In India, people consume a lot of sugar, but not much meat. They also have a low incidence of cancer.[3]

Although grains are acid forming, they neither cause nor promote cancer if grown organically. Whole grains have important fibers that promote healthy digestion, compared to meats, which contain no fiber to help push foods through the system. Whole grains with garden vegetables and sea vegetables, fresh green salads, and fruits should comprise the bulk of the diet—with vegetable, fruit, and herbal beverages taken between meals. Meat, fish, dairy, sweets, alcohol, and nuts should be kept to a minimum.

The morning after a dinner party where one has overindulged, it helps the system to eat plenty of oranges or fresh fruits to balance the acidity. Excellent teas for overacidity in the system are alfalfa, blessed thistle, buckthorn, dandelion, motherwort, mullein, red clover, watercress, and yarrow. If you crave sugar, try cutting down on salt intake and begin to replace foods containing refined white sugars with foods that contain "black" sugars such as date, malt, maple, and molasses. Black sugars are less acid-forming, and they contain alkaline-forming minerals and vitamins, which help in the combination of glucose in the body. Craving sugar can also be a sign to increase the protein in your diet. It is important to discourage children from sugary foods by giving them unsulfured dried fruits such as mango, pineapple, figs, papaya, raisins, banana chips, and other dried mixtures that can be purchased or can be made at home. If you use raisins, be sure they are organically grown since raisin crops are highly contaminated with pesticides. Dried foods travel well and maintain their nutritional quality, but they should be consumed within a year's time. Vitamins in pill form may cause acidity in the system if they are overused. Therefore, it is best to obtain nutrition from foods.

The famous Dr. Sagan Ishizuka, founder of Japanese Macrobiotic Medicine and Diet, believed that foods are the highest form of medicine. He divided foods into two activating categories: potassium and sodium. Potassium salt activates oxidation and sodium salt inhibits oxidation. Therefore, if one eats mostly grains and vegetables, which contain much potassium, the blood will oxidize well and allow better physiological functioning. On the other hand, if one eats more meat, poultry, fish, and eggs, which contain high amounts of sodium, blood oxidation is inhibited, leaving much poisonous acid. This is the reasoning behind the observation that when people balance these elements they live longer.

The Japanese custom is to cremate people when they die. It is believed that their ashes will be white if they ate a balanced diet, and black if they ate a lot of animal foods. This is how they can tell if a monk lived intelligently. In the United States we say, "You are what you eat."

BASIC ALKALINE-FORMING FOODS

Alkaline-forming foods should make up 75 to 85 percent of the diet. The following is a basic list of such foods. There is some inconsistency in the various charts and lists available, so I have listed these foods by using and combining all of the charts.

1. Fruits, including citrus (except cranberries, plums, prunes, and rhubarb).
2. Vegetables, particularly sea vegetables, mustard greens, parsley, and spinach.
3. Alkaline grains—millet, buckwheat, and sprouted grains.
4. Human milk, nonfat milk, goat's milk, all cheeses, plain yogurt, and egg yolks.
5. Tofu, soy sauce, and miso.
6. Coffee/tea.

7. Honey.

8. Spices and herbs (except garlic).

9. Mineral, soda, and well water.

10. Natural wines and sake (no sulfites or pesticides).

11. Almonds, brazil nuts, and all sprouted seeds.

12. Lima beans and sprouted beans.

BASIC ACID-FORMING FOODS

Acid-forming foods should make up 15 to 25 percent of the diet, depending upon lifestyle. If a person is more active, more fuel is needed than for a less active individual.

1. High protein foods, especially animal foods—meat, fish, dairy, and egg whites.

2. Brown rice, barley, wheat, oats, rye, corn, and breads.

3. Cashews, walnuts, peanuts, pecans, macadamias, and filberts.

4. Butter, cream, and nut oils.

5. Lentils, navy beans, kidney beans, and adzuki beans.

6. Alcoholic beverages and soft drinks.

7. White sugar and sugar substitutes, brown sugar, milk sugar, cane syrup, malt syrup, maple syrup, and molasses.

8. Cranberries, pomegranates, plums, prunes, and rhubarb.

9. Artificial and chemical additives and drugs.

FATS AND ACID-ALKALINE BALANCE

Fats are considered one of the three major nutrients. They also lubricate and cleanse. Fats are neutral in the system unless they are overused; then they create acidity in the body. There are two sources for fats: animal and vegetable.

Saturated fats come primarily from foods of animal origin—meat, poultry, whole milk, cream, butter, and cheese. They are also found in some vegetable oils such as coconut (90%), palm kernel (80%), palm (50%), and cottonseed (25%). After the age of thirty-five or forty, we begin to lose the ability to digest many fats well. Organic butter and cream are considered the best fats among these foods for digestibility, but they should be used sparingly; these milk fats can cause acidosis and lack of calcium in the body if overused. Clarified butter, called ghee, is highly valued in Ayurveda, the traditional natural healing system of India. Ghee is easy to digest and enhances absorption. Margarine is difficult to digest because it is usually hydrogenated, a process that turns oils into compounds essentially no different from saturated animal fats. Hydrogenated oils are present in many products and should be avoided. These fats promote arterial plaque, inhibit the production and efficient use of substances in the body that help the immune system, and reduce the body's ability to rid itself of carcinogens, drugs, and other toxins. Reading the labels of products helps us to avoid hydrogenated oils in processed foods—baked goods, potato chips, peanut butter, frozen dinners, candy, frozen foods, breads, margarines, and spray-on oils.

Polyunsaturated fats are contained in plant foods such as soybean, sunflower, safflower, walnut, almond, apricot, and corn oils, as well as in fish such as salmon and sardines. Sunflower oil offers a rich source of fatty acids and has no cholesterol. Walnut oil can be used like olive oil, but it has a short keeping time; therapeutically, it is useful in strengthening the liver and gallbladder. Omega-3, a highly polyunsaturated fat, has the greatest ability of all polyunsaturates to lower cholesterol levels.

Monounsaturated fats are found in poultry, peanuts, canola oil, avocado oil, and olive oil—which is the most concentrated source available. Studies have revealed that people who live in the Mediterranean area, where olive oil is traditionally used for cooking, have a lower incidence of heart disease than North Americans. Olive oil also stimulates clearing of the liver and gallbladder. Canola, olive, and grapeseed oils hold up the best when heated, so these oils are best for cooking. However, no food is healthful if fried in overheated oil. If the oil smokes when heated, begin again and use a lower temperature. Canola oil, extracted from the tiny rapeseed, is popular in Canada and the Far East. It has the lowest saturated fat content of all commonly used vegetable oils. Canola oil's monounsaturated oleic acids also help keep it from becoming rancid. All oils should be stored in a cool dark place or refrigerated.

SELECTING THE BEST FATS

The key to selecting the best dietary fats to promote health, cleanse, and reduce your body's toxin load, lies in the type of fatty acids contained in the various foods and oils consumed. The endocrine gland network is responsible for production of the hormones that promote youthfulness for body and mind. These glands, along with the arteries, are subject to accumulations of the nonbeneficial cholesterol deposits caused by an excessive intake of hard, saturated, overheated fats. These fats inhibit the rhythm and efficiency of the glands, which, in turn, stresses the overall health of the whole body.

The use of unsaturated and cold-pressed seed oils will help clean the "rust" from the body's network of glands and promote healing by supplying essential fatty acids, which the body cannot produce on its own. All vegetable oils contain fatty acids. The two essential fatty acids, omega-3 and omega-6, which the body cannot produce, fight damage caused by toxic chemicals and help keep our immune systems strong. They must be supplied in the diet.

These oils are important in our diet because omega-3 contains linolenic acid, which the body metabolizes into prostaglandins. These substances resemble hormones and regulate white blood cells in the immune system, particularly B- and T-cells. The B-cells produce antibodies to destroy toxic invaders, and T-cells alert our body when the invaders have been vanquished. These cells are antibody producers and so the inability to make prostaglandins properly impairs immune function and increases our vulnerability to toxic chemicals.

Because of the scarcity in the American diet of omega-3 fatty acids, it is likely that millions are deficient in this essential nutrient. Signs of an omega-3 fatty acid deficiency include allergies, dry hair and skin, rashes or tiny bumps on the back of the arms, and brittle nails. Good sources of omega-3 are fresh flaxseed oil, which contains 57 percent omega-3 fatty acids, and hempseed oil. These are easily added to salad dressings and can be combined with other oils for delicious flavor. Flaxseed oil is found mainly in the refrigerated section of natural foods stores. Whole flaxseeds are inexpensive and add a wholesome, nutty flavor to foods. Keep them in the refrigerator and grind them fresh. Add freshly ground flaxseed to your morning oatmeal, juice, fresh fruit, pancakes, rolls, and breads. Flaxseed and hempseed oils are not inexpensive but are worth the benefits. Hempseed oil is rich in both omega-3 and omega-6 fatty acids. It is more stable than flaxseed oil. Hempseed oil has a pleasant, nutty taste, similar to sunflower oil, which makes it a perfect salad oil. This raw, unrefined oil should be refrigerated, and it can be frozen to extend shelf life. See Sources.

Pumpkin seed oil has 15 percent omega-3 fatty acids, and canola oil, made from the rapeseed, has 10 percent. In Japan, rapeseed oil is valued for cooking in some villages. (They also eat the rape—from the mustard family—as a vegetable in spring, boiling the tender shoots and immature seed heads as potherbs.) Other oils containing omega-3 fatty acids in smaller amounts are English walnut, avocado, wheat germ, and olive.

The oil from all fish contains the valuable omega-3, but cold-water fish oil from mackerel, tuna, trout, herring, salmon, sturgeon, whitefish, anchovy, eel, and halibut has the greatest concentrations. Algae, seaweed, and the plants in plankton form also contain omega-3.

Though soybeans contain a great amount of omega-3, commercially produced soybean oil does not represent a good source of it. Because linolenic (omega-3) oils oxidize rapidly and spoil easily, soybean oil manufacturers try to decrease the risk of spoilage by removing these acids. However, soybeans, navy, great northern, and kidney beans are good sources of essential omega-3 fatty acids.

Choose oils made from organically grown crops and that are expeller- or cold-pressed. Expeller-pressing means that the oil source—such as corn—has been mashed for the oil; this process leaves the oil much purer than that produced through solvent methods. Use virgin and extra virgin olive oils, which are made from the first pressings of the olives. "Pure" olive oil is often extracted with chemical solvents. Since oils should be used sparingly in the diet, it is important that the ones we choose be the best available. Cold-pressed organic vegetable and seed oils such as safflower, flaxseed, hempseed, sunflower, corn, wheat, and those from other seed-bearing plants work with minerals to establish a balanced hormone rhythm that works to improve body metabolism. The adrenal glands are soothed and refreshed, as well as nourished, by the intake of these seed oils.

Rancid oil is dangerous because it is highly reactive and inhibits nutrient absorption in the body. Heat, light, and air are destructive to oils. It is best to buy small amounts at a time and store the oils in the refrigerator or a cool place away from direct sunlight. Some people add vitamin E to oils to retard oxidation. Vitamin E is a natural antioxidant and helpful to your body in metabolizing unsaturated fats. Add about 200 units of vitamin E to a 16-ounce bottle of oil when you open it. Repeat in a few weeks until the oil is consumed. Flaxseed oil is not good for frying, but it can be used for baking. Always gently heat oils when they are called for in cooking and use heat-stable oils such as olive, canola, and grapeseed. These oils do not form cancer-stimulating free radicals unless they are heated above 400 degrees. Deep-fried foods are dangerous because the fats are intensely heated and are usually saturated or hydrogenated.

Choosing the best fats for the diet is as important to our bodies as vitamins and minerals; how we use them makes the difference in whether we are healthy or unhealthy. The skin and hair of people who keep good fats and oils out of their diet are excessively dry, flaky, lifeless, and lusterless. (Very low-fat, low-calorie diets can also cause gallstones.) The good fats and oils are not only essential to maintain health, they are also important for maintaining beauty, youth, and vigor!

THE KEY TO CHOLESTEROL

The current of blood in our body is unbelievably strong, rushing with the turbulence of the swiftest mountain streams. But while the banks of the mountain stream are altered by erosion, the body tissues are unaffected by the violent currents of blood. How is this possible? Protection is afforded by the lubrication of the lining of the arterial walls. Nature has perfected a frictionless substance that keeps the body from being washed away by its own blood currents. The key element of this most effective lubrication is a fat-like substance called cholesterol.

The idea that a high-fat diet is necessarily harmful to the arteries is contradicted by a careful study of the diet of Eskimos. Their bones are stronger than those of any other culture, their strength is prodigious, and their health is phenomenal. Although on a high-fat diet—and a so-called "saturated" fat intake at that—their blood cholesterol is normal and their arteries are perfect. They consume fats that are not overly heated or processed, and their bodies quickly utilize the fats in the extreme cold.

Question: What fats are healthful for the body? Answer: Natural and unadulterated fats. Animal fats—meat, organ, marrow, and brain fats. Vegetable fats in beans, seeds, nuts, and avocados. Bananas and tropical fruit including papaya, mango, sapote, and coconut. As far as their usefulness to the body, it makes little difference whether they are saturated or unsaturated, provided the liver is healthy enough to synthesize them for food.

Fats, saturated or unsaturated, are most harmful to the body when they are used as shortening or cooking oil, that is, when they are heated with other foods, especially the starches. Fried bread or potatoes, doughnuts, hot cakes, pie crust, cakes, and pastries all contain altered cholesterol. When you eat these highly regarded confections, the result is degraded artery lining, erosion of the arteries, and atherosclerosis. The greatest offenders are french fries, doughnuts, potato chips, and popcorn (if the popcorn is "popped" in cooking oil). The surest way to render cooked string beans or other vegetables indigestible is to saturate or "season" them with bacon grease.

The resulting cholesterol is used by the body for arterial lining, but being an unnatural or altered cholesterol, it fails to wear well, soon breaks down, and is corroded; this results in various forms of arterial disease and degeneration—arteriosclerosis (commonly called hardening or narrowing of the artery walls, which causes them to lose their elasticity); atherosclerosis (fatty deposits on the arterial walls, which may impede or block the blood flow); coronary thrombosis (blood clotting in the arteries, which blocks the blood supply to the heart); and aneurism (ruptured abnormality in artery wall). In these states the concentration of cholesterol in the blood is much higher than the normal level. Even if every trace of cholesterol is omitted from the diet, it continues to circulate in the blood, for the liver manufactures it; our bodies require it.

EGGS

The majority of eggs consumed by humans come from the chicken, and yet chicken eggs are very much misunderstood in the United States. This may be because eggs were proclaimed hazardous to health by the American Heart Association, owing to the cholesterol content in their yolks. However, current research finds that the choline and lecithin contained in egg yolk actually "cause" the high-density lipoproteins, which in turn break up the unnatural cholesterol and help keep arteries clean.

Egg yolk is a source of complete protein. The value of any protein depends upon the number and amount of essential amino acids it contains. Proteins containing the eight essential amino acids in generous amounts are called "complete" or "adequate." These essential amino acids are supplied in greatest abundance in the egg yolk.

Egg yolk is one important food that offers help for cell rebuilding and tissue regeneration. Vitamins A, B_1 (thiamine), B_2 (riboflavin), B_5, B_6, B_{12}, D, and E and the minerals magnesium, phosphorus, selenium, and sulphur, are found in the rich yolk of the egg. The abundance of lecithin in the yolk (14% more than in cholesterol) is of great importance to every cell and organ in the human system.

While lecithin is found in every living cell, its highest concentration is in the vital organs—the brain, the heart, the liver, and the kidneys. Our brains show a dry composition of 30 percent lecithin. It performs an astonishing range of vital functions directly affecting our health and well-being. Lecithin is found in plant life as seeds, in yeast and soybeans, but it is most abundant in organically raised, fertile eggs. It is one of the most important nutrients to be consumed when one is under stress—to restore nerve energies. Lecithin granules may be used to supplement the diet. Read the label with care. If choline chloride is listed as an ingredient, avoid this synthetic product and look instead for one that contains natural phosphatidyl choline, which is body-building, tissue-regenerating "true" lecithin.

Egg yolk is utilized creatively in food preparation throughout Europe, Africa, and Asia in ways rarely seen in the West. Throughout France and Spain, simple vegetable casseroles are topped with raw egg yolk after being baked. Egg yolk is added while the dish is hot so that the gentle heat delicately cooks the outer edges of the yolk. In Africa, raw egg yolk crowns the various vegetable and meat tagines to be lightly cooked before the delicious tagine is enjoyed.

Tibetan lamas eat one raw egg yolk before or after a meal because they know that the yolk contains half of the sixteen elements required by the brain, nerves, blood, and tissues. The lamas would not eat whole eggs unless they were engaged in hard manual labor because the egg whites are used only by the muscles.

In the United States, the FDA recommends that eggs be thoroughly cooked before serving to kill any bacterial contamination that may cause illness. The very young, the elderly, pregnant women, and those already weakened by serious illness, or whose immune systems are weakened, should not eat raw eggs or any foods prepared with raw eggs.

SUGAR

Chemically refined white sugar creates an acid condition in the system and will tend to leave a harsh "residue" on the glands, affecting hormonal balance and impeding the healthful function of the hormones. An excessive amount of refined sugar also speeds up body metabolism, causing overwork by the glandular system and contributing to internal exhaustion. Processed white sugar literally leaches certain substances out of the body—it requires energy and metabolic substances pulled from the body's bank deposit of nutrients to digest it. It takes more energy to get rid of it than it gives. It is truly a thief of potent proportions. A good way to think of refined white sugar, especially as we are ingesting it each day, is as an antinutrient. However, do not throw away your white sugar. It is useful for the Mediterranean Oil Bath (p. 203) and for making Kombucha Tea (p. 219).

All types of sugar should be used sparingly. If overused, processed honey in particular can produce various complications, especially if it is heated. Cooking alters its attributes and makes it incompatible with the body. Heated honey can clog the digestive tract and create toxins. The Russians have studied people in their country who have lived past 100 years of age. Many were found to be poor beekeepers who supplemented their diet with the "dirty" honey that collected at the bottom of the hives. This honey still contained the royal jelly, bee pollen, vitamins, and minerals that make honey a highly valuable food when raw and unheated. (Maple syrup and molasses are better suited for heated or baked dishes.)

Other popular sugars, Rapadura and Sucanat, are made by pressing ripe sugar cane to extract the juice and then evaporating the moisture, conserving the vitamins and minerals present in the cane. Only molasses has more vitamins and minerals per serving of sweetener. Danish scientists have developed a natural sweetener named Fructan derived from the Jerusalem artichoke. This new sweetener is low in calories and stabilizes blood sugar levels. All these sweeteners offer high-quality alternatives to refined white sugar. The flavor of the dishes you make with them is enriched, not overwhelmed by a too sweet taste.

The daily craving for sugar is generally caused by imbalance and dietary deficiency. Cutting down on salt intake and adding more complete protein dishes to the diet are recommended by naturopathic physicians for those craving sugar. When cleansing fasts are incorporated into the diet, the body begins to purify and to balance chemically; it then becomes less congested, allowing for improved absorption of vitamins and minerals. When the body is well-nourished, many cravings vanish.

HORMONES AND YOUR HEALTH

Our bodies are run by hormones that balance bodily systems throughout our lifetime. Hormonal balance is an important factor in maintaining good health, and the right diet plays a large part in providing the nutrients needed by the body to produce its own natural hormones in both men and women.

If we are constantly stressed by lack of proper nutrition or physical or emotional factors, hormonal imbalance may occur. The level of hormones slowly declines as we age, but scientific research shows a more pronounced decline of natural hormones in nonhealthy groups, especially in high-cardiovascular-risk groups. Nutritional support of the glands that balance our hormonal levels is very important for women and men, particularly those over forty years of age.

Hormone therapy involving animal-derived and synthetic drugs is coming under increasing scrutiny because of possible health risks and side effects. The nutrients needed to make both male and female hormones are the same. When the body makes its own hormones with the help of certain nutrient supportive foods, there are no side effects. Many foods such as flaxseed, peas, and soybeans contain hormone-like components called sterols, which can have a beneficial effect on natural hormone production in the body. However, it is the essential fatty acids—in which many people have a deficiency—that provide the phytosterols required by the glands for proper hormonal balance. Phytosterols are derived from the unrefined oils of rice bran, wheat germ, safflower, soybeans, flaxseed, and hempseed. The oils must be consumed in their raw form, cold-pressed, and without alteration from cooking or exposure to light and oxygen. When essential fatty acids are deficient, we can expect a plethora of health problems ranging from fatigue to lack of sexual energy.

FOOD COMBINING IS A LIFESTYLE

Throughout history there is recorded evidence of the compatibility of food groups. There are laws relating to food combining mentioned in the Bible and other ancient texts. In recent years, food combining has been developed into a science by Doctor W. H. Hay and others, such as the late Edgar Cayce.

The reasoning behind combining certain foods is based on electromagnetic energy. Our food has electromagnetic power or energy, and every living body has an electromagnetic force field; the higher the force field frequency, the healthier the body. The lower the frequency, the more the body needs help to generate this energy because we feel low in energy. The electromagnetic force field, also called the "aura," is a protective layer around the body and around each organ; it gives protection against all kinds of intruders. Every food has the ability to increase or decrease your energy level. Food combining develops and ensures a healthy digestion, so that what we eat can release its electromagnetic force and feed the protective shield around us, providing optimal nourishment.

1. Basically, combining foods "well" means separating protein meals from carbohydrate meals, because grains and animal protein eaten at the same meal completely counteract the electromagnetic energy. Rice is the only exception; it hinders the flow, but does not neutralize it entirely. This means

   A. no bread with eggs.

   B. no bread with sausage or meat.

   C. no bread with cheese.

   D. no grains with fruit juice; they build mucus in the stomach and negate the energy patterns.

   E. no white bread, potatoes, pasta, or any two foods of such nature in the same meal.

2. Vegetables that develop above the ground, when combined with grains, offer the highest form of electromagnetic energy, and the body responds to them with a buoyant, contented feeling.

3. Vegetables that develop above the ground, when combined with protein, also become a high form of electromagnetic energy for the body.

4. Vegetables that develop below the ground (root vegetables), when combined with protein—meat with potatoes and carrots—offer a fair amount of energies.

5. Milk does not combine well with any type of meat, be it fish, fowl, red or white meat; but cream may be used with meats. Milk neutralizes the stomach acidity, but meats require strong acidity to be digested. Meats combined with milk will remain in the stomach and putrefy, which creates a complete void in the electromagnetic pattern. Do not take milk or cream in coffee or caffeinated tea.

6. The various types of meat should not be mixed together. Red meat, poultry, fish, shellfish, and "white" meat such as pork should be eaten separately, not combined with one another.

7. The most digestible fats are butter, cream, and olive oil. Avoid fried foods of any kind.

8. Fruits and vegetables should be eaten at separate meals. Fruit is best eaten by itself at breakfast or as a snack. Melons and citrus in particular should be eaten alone. The only exception to this law is apples, which can be combined with vegetable salads, grains, and proteins without neutralizing electromagnetic energy.

The finer points regarding the art of food combining are illustrated in the following chart.

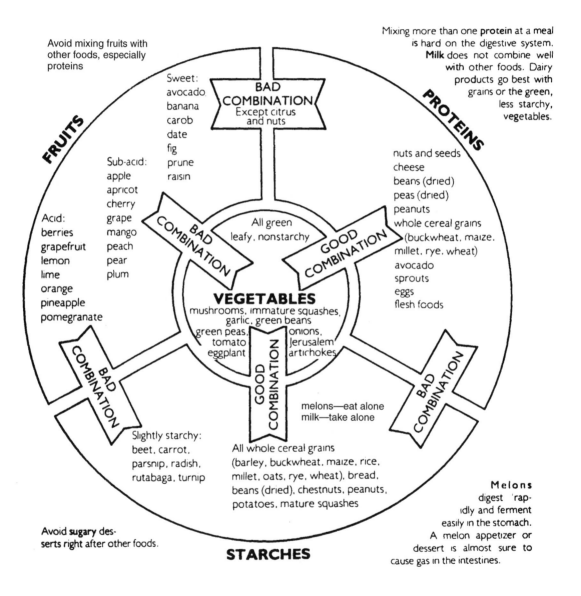

A scientific set of instructions as founded by the Natural Hygiene Institute and Herbert Shelton for nonfermenting properly digesting food combinations.

DIGESTION

Diet is the plan of what to eat. Nutrition is the study of what happens to the food in the body after it is eaten. Assimilation is an individual's capacity to utilize the food and the body's management of the complicated metabolic processes of digestion, absorption, and elimination.

It is estimated that 80 percent of people in the United States have digestive disorders of one form or another. We are nourished only in proportion to what we are able to digest and assimilate. Digestion is a very important factor in achieving and maintaining health; through the ages people have utilized the powers of certain foods to enhance and stimulate this process. The body heals itself through proper absorption of quality foods.

The body is a physical masterpiece, often able to endure up to forty to fifty years of dietary abuse before the organs begin to break down. If the food we consume (white sugar, soda, alcohol, coffee, refined flour and grain, overcooked foods, and so forth) consistently contains little or no nutritional value, the body must expend precious energy in the form of vitamins, minerals, and enzymes trying to assimilate nutrients that do not exist. If our eating habits are geared to stimulate the life force of our being—eating to live, instead of living to eat—our bodies will safely see us through what "should" be the most pleasant, productive, and powerful times of our lives—the middle to later years.

All cells and tissues in the body need nourishment, and each part may be subject to nutrition that is faulty in varying degrees. It is possible that imperfect nutrition may be a basic cause of most of the noninfectious diseases—ones that at present are poorly diagnosed and controlled by medical science. If our body cells are ailing, as they must be in disease, the chances are excellent that it is because they are being inadequately provisioned.

In the processing of foods by the body, a series of digestions occurs, beginning with the action of enzymes in the mouth. This action creates heat, slight though it may be, and to this heat is added that of friction, caused by the grinding of the food by the teeth. When the food goes into the stomach, another cooking occurs—the heat of hydrochloric acid. Each of these heatings changes the nature of the food. If one lacks the proper levels of enzymes in the mouth, or fails to chew the food sufficiently, or has hydrochloric acid deficiency in the stomach, then digestion will be impaired from the start.

The latest research in microbiology confirms what has been known for centuries. One example concerns the advice to take a "small" amount of sea salt *before* beginning a meal. This seems to be contradicted by modern medical wisdom, which stresses the harmful effects of excess salt consumption. We are not adding the salt directly to food or cooking with salt for flavor, because using salt in this way can destroy much of the vitamins in foods, but we are taking a small amount on an empty stomach "before" eating a meal. A knowledge of the metabolism of the body illustrates the wisdom of this suggestion. The salt is composed of two chemicals: sodium and chloride. Harmful effects of excess salt are primarily associated with raised levels of sodium, not chlorides. In fact people who eliminate sea salt entirely from their diet may be subject to further disease, caused by lack of proper levels of hydrochloric acid.

The chlorides present in salt constitute the only readily available source of chlorides with which the body can manufacture hydrochloric acid, which is vital for proper digestion in the stomach. Thus, taking salt before a meal allows any deficiency of hydrochloric acid to be made up just before introducing new food. If we use sea salt correctly—and moderately—it is beautifying to the skin, giving it a soft glow, but excessive use causes the skin to itch. Salt also stimulates the appetite.

Salt is a necessary ingredient in the preparation of certain foods. The macrobiotic sea salt mined and sold by Niguro Miramoto is considered the best in the world. Read the label carefully on any salt to find one that does not contain sugar (or dextrose), which is the main adulterant in many salts sold in stores.

DIGESTIVE AIDS

At about age twenty-five, the body begins to lose digestive power through the dissipation of hydrochloric acid. After age forty, we should begin helping the digestion with food enzymes, eating more live foods before meals—such as papaya, avocado, mint, ginger, aloe vera juice, anise, and sea salt to help digestion. Ground fennel seed and ginger mixed with honey is a specific remedy for all cases of poor digestion; this has been handed down from the time of Hippocrates.

Research on enzyme activity in food digestion proves that 80 percent of enzyme activity is devoted to the digestion of the food we eat. Since all enzymes contained in raw foods are destroyed by freezing, boiling, frying, and radiation, many people consume food that has no enzyme content whatsoever. When spices such as ginger, turmeric, cumin, and cinnamon—the heating spices—are consumed, the production of digestive enzymes by the body increases dramatically. Whenever the body undergoes fasting, enzymes normally assigned to digest food are freed to conduct healing functions, such as dissolving latent tumors.

A mixture of $1/4$ cup aloe vera juice, $1/4$ cup pure water, and $1/2$ cup papaya puree is delicious and soothing to the digestive organs. Interchange these with peppermint

INGREDIENTS	AMOUNT
aloe vera juice	$1/4$ C.
pure water	$1/4$ C.
papaya puree	$1/2$ C.

and orange rind or ginger with lemon and maple syrup teas. These are greatly appreciated and enjoyed by all, and they are good to serve about 30 minutes before or after a meal. Drinking liquids such as alcohol, coffee, juices, sodas, teas, and ice water just before and during a meal will dilute and weaken the digestive forces of the body greatly.

We all recognize how important relaxation is to digestion. If we eat when we are tired, angry, excited, under stress or other strong emotions, the most nutritious food will give us indigestion; and, if we make a habit of it, ultimately we may get an ulcer. Avoid eating foods that disagree with you and work at developing your instincts for what your body tells you it needs. Allow your food to cool before eating and stop eating before you are too full. One of the easiest ways to destroy a good meal is to overstuff and overtax your digestive system.

When the digestion in the stomach is finished, the food is a semifluid mass called chyme—the essence of the food. The stomach sends this chyme via the small intestine (where additional enzymes create added heat and processing) to the liver. At the liver, the finest parts are made into blood, and valuable micronutrient components are carried out into the general system to participate in various chemical processes that transform them into the myriad forms of the body. The evacuation of waste products from the large intestine is the final processing of completely metabolized food.

The Chinese, Ayurvedic, Hippocratic, Galenic, Arabic, and Hebraic medical and health systems all teach that the *single* most important factor for complete digestion is that foods must contain sufficient metabolic heat. They state that food that is cold in its essence has a net effect of lowering metabolism, and that the origin of every disease is cold. All elements of Nature can be assigned a value according to this system of heating and cooling effects, and the diet can be adjusted according to season, climate, altitude, prevalent illness, and so forth. For thousands of years, this system has been developed and refined. It is based on two notions: the four bodily essences or humors (blood, phlegm, yellow bile, black bile) and the effect of heating and cooling foods.

We can see that the basic diet of the majority of North Americans—milk, beef, potatoes, lettuce salads, refined white sugar and flour products, cheese, butter, margarine—is all cold food. Cold foods in excess lead to imbalance of the phlegm humor, helping to cause the list of complaints that are epidemic in this country: migraine headaches, menstrual cramps, lung and chest problems, arthritis, constipation. As we continue to choose our food poorly, the other humors—blood, yellow bile, and black bile—become imbalanced in time. When such imbalance reaches the fourth stage of black bile humor, diseases such as cancer, arteriosclerosis, and emphysema arise.

Consider some of the items from the heating foods list—lamb, liver, goat, ghee, beet, lentils, eggplant, chickpeas, dried fruits, nuts, honey, and the spices such as cardamom, fenugreek, ginger, cumin, saffron, and cinnamon. We observe that these are among some of the least consumed foods in the United States. If they are eaten, it is usually as part of some exotic experimental cuisine, but not as part of the daily diet.

Heating foods are necessary for the body to achieve and maintain a complete metabolic digestion of foods. When it is indicated that a food is heating or hot, it does not mean hot to the taste, nor does this refer to its caloric value. Rather, *a heating food is one that creates a net effect in the body of promoting metabolism.* Balancing the heating foods and the cooling foods will greatly aid digestion and is a most elegant, useful, and refined manner of constructing a diet. If followed with sincerity, it will provide a good basis of health for people of all ages.

All spices, and many herbs, encourage the flow of digestive juices and discourage stomach spasms and flatulence. These good properties are entirely due to the essential oils they contain. The better your food tastes and smells, the more you enjoy it and the better you digest it. However, if you take too many spicy foods, you may overstrain your digestion and burden your kidneys; in moderation spices aid digestion.

Moderation should ever be the golden rule in the diet. A meal of many courses and heavy food throws a sudden load on the heart, which then is obliged to pump an extra supply of blood to digest it. Frequent small meals are better than overeating at any one meal or alternating between feast and famine. Sweet desserts and fatty foods, including fatty meats and gravies, should give way to vegetable soup, lean meats, vegetables, salads, and fruits.

WATER

The water presently on our planet has been constantly recirculated since it was formed some 4.3 billion years ago. It is the same water that coursed through the veins of the dinosaurs and of your ancestors. It is wise to take responsibility for the purity of your water. Learn about your water supply, so you will be aware of potential problems. It is a good idea to have your water tested; if the test shows pesticides, pollutants, radiation, or other dangers, a water filter system will be a life-saving supplement to your home.

The independent and respected National Sanitation Foundation of East Lansing, Michigan, certifies which home filter systems deliver on their claims, providing an NSF seal of approval only to systems that meet the foundation's highest standards. Another institute with information about filtration systems is the Water Quality Association of Lisle, Illinois. It also guarantees performance standards for its members' products. Their information will help you decide which water filter to purchase. They will send you general information about water quality problems and point-of-use technologies that can be used in the home or office. See Sources.

WATER TESTING

Firms that can test your water for lead, bacteria, metal, minerals, nitrates, pesticides, and industrial solvents are listed in the back of this book. Costs range from around $30 to over $200 for a most comprehensive test. See Sources.

OTHER WATER HAZARDS

Boiling water before use will not always make it safe for drinking or cooking. Boiling water kills off bacteria, but it does not remove many heavy metals and other toxic chemicals such as lead, asbestos, copper, and trihalomethanes (carcinogenic by-products of chlorination). Boiling can actually concentrate harmful substances in the water left after evaporation. This means that even water labeled "distilled" could still be contaminated. Run tap water for several minutes before use to flush out lead, and buy a quality home water filter to remove other substances, as commercial bottled waters could possibly have the same contaminants.

ALCOHOLIC BEVERAGES

Alcohol was not considered evil or inherently unhealthy by the ancient sages; indeed, wine was used in ancient practice to dispel fatigue and enhance digestion, and there are detailed descriptions of alcoholic preparations for healing included in the classic texts. Moderation and appropriateness were considered important since alcohol was acknowledged to badly aggravate the system when used to excess, especially in the summer. Like other substances, it is recommended that alcohol be utilized with respect and awareness.

Throughout history, and all around the world, wine has played an integral part in religious celebrations and worship, and this intimate association of wine with religion was carried over to the North American colonies. Wine continues into the present as a central element in ceremonies, and it is shared among groups of friends for an aesthetic experience of enjoying fine food and drink. Wine, it seems, is intimately associated with our spiritual heritage and, in moderation, helps us to celebrate the most blessed things in life.

It is well known, however, that even moderate drinking can increase the waistline and that heavy drinking over age forty accelerates the body's natural declines in testosterone level and liver efficiency.

The ancient Romans were well aware that the use of alcohol could poison a fetus before birth and contaminate the mother's milk after birth. Accordingly, alcoholic drinks were prohibited by law to a Roman mother while an infant was dependent upon her for support.

Present-day scientific research suggests that there are beneficial effects to small amounts of alcohol, taken daily, which help to reduce cholesterol in the blood and circulatory system. The largest amount of alcohol which can be taken daily, without producing poisonous effects and serious consequences, is 1½ ounces. Conversely, the overuse of alcohol is one of the most potent influences in increasing our susceptibility to disease. Alcohol is a powerful antiseptic and has the effect of hardening tissues. An apple or the body of an animal placed in alcoholic fluid cannot undergo decomposition.

Experiments have shown that the efficiency of the kidneys in eliminating poisons is diminished by nearly one-half when we ingest large quantities of alcohol; the body temperature drops, muscular strength is decreased, digestion is inhibited, the nerves are paralyzed so that they lose their normal sensibility, and judgment is impaired.

The potent carcinogen urethane is present in many brands of alcoholic beverages, including wine. Drinking urethane-contaminated alcohol presents high risk for cancer even in moderate drinkers. The kinds of alcoholic beverages most likely to be tainted with very high concentrations of urethane are straight American bourbon whiskeys, European fruit brandies, cream sherries, port wines, Japanese sakes, Chinese wines, and European liqueurs. Rums have moderately low levels of urethane. Tequilas have very low levels, as do beer and malt beverages. Vodkas have virtually no urethane and have low pesticide levels.

Grape table wines vary in the level of urethane but in general they contain low levels. However, nonorganic wines have extremely elevated concentrations of pesticides. To qualify as a top quality product, wines must be pesticide-free! Fortunately, there is a movement in the wine industry to do just that. Since Roman times, sulfur has been added to wine to remove unwanted yeast and bacteria, and to stabilize flavor and color. Because some 0.4 percent of the population is severely allergic to sulfites, according to the U.S. Food and Drug Administration estimates, the government requires wines containing more than 10 parts per million (ppm) to carry the label: "Contains sulfites." Strict standards are also set by the California Certified Organic Farmers group. Sulfite usage by responsible wine-makers is minuscule.

Sulfites are, in fact, a natural by-product of the wine fermentation process, even if sulfur is not added. Sulfites are naturally occurring in wine due to fermenting yeasts present on grape skins, generating amounts ranging from 6 to 40 ppm. There is no such thing as a sulfite-free wine; therefore, people who are allergic to sulfites should not drink wine.

Currently in the United States there are more than a dozen organic wine producers. In France there are some 250 certified organic wine producers, many of whom export to the United States. The list of organic wine producers (see Sources) will assist those who wish to secure healthful wines for celebration, ceremony, and simple pleasure.

MILK

In Biblical times, refrigeration did not exist, so the milk had to be used fresh, immediately after each milking. After 24 hours, a considerable change occurs in which milk becomes much less compatible with the body. After 3 days of aging, the milk is completely incompatible with the body and can cause problems. Some of it can enter the arteries, attaching itself to the walls in the form of sludge or shellac, and mucus can be generated in the intestines, contaminating the entire body.

Milk processed under current conditions reaches the home or the grocery shelf 3 days old or older. It has been pasteurized and homogenized, and a considerable number of products may have been added to it. The substance sold as milk simply bears little resemblance to the natural food, and it cannot be expected to be properly processed by the body.

If clean raw milk can be obtained and consumed within 24 hours of milking, it can be an excellent food for many people. However, some people may suffer mucous production from raw milk, and others may not have the proper enzymes to digest the substance. If milk is not tolerated by a person, it should not be used.

Raw milk is always heated before serving to kill bacteria and make it easier to digest. Spices such as cinnamon, cardamom, ginger, and black peppercorns are delicious added to the heated milk. Herbal teas such as peppermint and ginger are also a pleasing addition to milk.

One 8-ounce glass of raw milk is adequate for most people to consume in one day. If fresh organic raw milk is not available for daily use, there are substitutes that produce very good results in cooking and baking and provide optimal nutrients for the body. These are as follows: cultured buttermilk, kefir milk, coconut milk, heavy cream, dried milk, oat milk, rice milk, soy milk, nut milk, and yogurt. All of these may be diluted with water or apple juice to thin or stretch the ingredients depending on the desired effect or taste you wish to achieve.

Goat's milk is more astringent and less mucus-forming than cow's milk; it is often well-absorbed by individuals sensitive to cow's milk. Its high buffering capacity makes it useful for calming and healing stomach ulcers. In ancient times, goat's milk was used in India to stimulate milk production in nursing mothers. Goat cheese is easy to digest.

Sheep's milk and buffalo milk are rare in the diet of today. Sheep's milk has been known for its excellent calming properties, and buffalo milk was recommended by Ayurvedic healers for its excellent ability to induce sleep.

Soy milk does not contain the bacteria found in animal milks, and it can be a good alternative if from organically grown beans. Like most high-protein foods, it promotes building, not cleansing. It is best used in restorative and maintenance programs, and can be warmed with cinnamon, cardamom, nutmeg, or ginger. Dried soy milk powder and soy protein powder are much more difficult to digest than the whole liquid soy milks.

❧ HOT SPICED MILKS

Gently warm all ingredients—do not boil—in a small glass or stainless-steel pot for 15 minutes or more. Strain and enjoy.

INGREDIENTS	AMOUNT
milk (raw), oat or soy milk	1 C.
pure water	1 C.
cardamom (powdered)	$^1/_4$ tsp.
ginger (powdered)	$^1/_4$ tsp.
cloves (powdered)	$^1/_4$ tsp.
caraway seed	$^1/_4$ tsp.

❧ HOT MILK WITH NUTMEG

Gently warm milk, but do not boil; remove from heat and stir in nutmeg. Cover and steep for 5 minutes, strain. This is a good drink for calming the nerves or relieving insomnia.

INGREDIENTS	AMOUNT
milk (raw)	1 C.
nutmeg (ground)	$^1/_2$ tsp.

❧ HOT GINGER MILK

Gently heat all ingredients, except the ghee. Remove from heat and steep for 5 minutes. Strain, then stir in ghee.

INGREDIENTS	AMOUNT
cow's or goat's milk (raw)	1 C.
pure water	1 C.
freshly grated gingerroot	1 tsp.
cardamom seed	3 or 4
ghee (clarified butter)	$^1/_2$ tsp.

COOKING UTENSILS

Take a close look at your cooking implements. The best cooks are alert and aware of the important role quality cooking utensils play in food preparation. There are many creative and elegantly simple natural materials that are utilized in cooking: the bamboo steamer, banana leaves, corn husks, woven palms, sturdy branches, and parchment paper to name a few. These are all benign compared to the modern metals that are generally used today. The various metals react chemically with foods and may affect the quality of the best ingredients. There are hidden dangers in aluminum cookware in particular. If the food is overdone, waterlogged, or burned, any food value is lost through destruction of life-giving vitamins, minerals, and the live food enzymes contained in the raw foods that are meant to nourish the body.

Aluminum Cookware: Aluminum is constantly used in our society as cookware, in lining containers, and added to some deodorant products and certain antacids. However, aluminum is a toxic mineral and should never be used as a cooking utensil or ingested in any form. Many restaurants and commercial food preparation systems use aluminum pots, tins, and foils to prepare, store, and cook foods. When food is prepared in aluminum, a reaction occurs causing the aluminum to displace any of the other metal minerals the food may contain such as iron, zinc, chrome, magnesium, copper, or manganese, all of which are precious to the body. The food may then taste metallic because it contains aluminum and is poisonous. Aluminum in all forms should be avoided; this includes the use of aluminum foil to wrap or cook food in. Aluminum cookware is easily bent out of shape, it pits, discolors, and reacts with both acidic and alkaline foods.

Once ingested, aluminum remains in the body permanently unless some method is used to eliminate the poison. Aluminum seems to settle in weak spots in the body; it causes severe stress to the cells and prevents rebuilding. Cells touched by aluminum degenerate so that a small area within the body may become dysfunctional or die. It is slow acting and may not create a health problem for years after ingestion. People with joint disorders and back deterioration and Alzheimer's patients have been found to have an abundance of aluminum deposited in the body.

Adverse effects on vitality are possible from residing in aluminum homes, trailers, or campers. Carefully analyze your environment to determine all possible sources of contact with aluminum. Body products, medicines, and drugs may contain aluminum.

Teflon Cookware: Teflon itself is a toxic substance, and if it is scraped off, it can become mixed with the food and ingested. Teflon pots are often aluminum pots coated with teflon.

Enamel Pots: Enamel pots often contain cadmium, which also is a toxic metal. Never use an enamel pot if it has been chipped or has cracks in the enamel.

Earthen Cookware: Care should be taken in using earthen pots due to the possibility of the clay containing toxic substances. Glazed earthen designs often have high levels of lead in them that may cause acute illnesses.

Copper Cookware: The Romans used copper kettles as cooking utensils, and in doing so poisoned themselves. Copper-poisoned people have a burning sensation in the throat and tonsils, and some have it throughout the system. Copper easily settles in the brain, and it accumulates in the ovaries of women. Therefore, *unlined* copper cookware is not recommended for food preparation. Copper conducts and diffuses heat better than any other metal commonly used for cookware, so it is lined with stainless steel for our protection. When buying copper pans look for heavy-gauge, well-made pans with handles made from a different metal and sturdily riveted.

Stainless-Steel Cookware: Stainless steel is made of iron and chrome, both of which the body can absorb healthfully. Stainless-steel cookware may be used in the safe preparation of foods; it is extremely durable, totally nonreactive, and noncorrodible. But, because stainless steel does not conduct and diffuse heat efficiently, it is usually joined to more conductive metals such as copper or aluminum. Many other combinations are possible—pans often have 5- and even 7-ply construction. Stainless steel is less expensive than copper, it is easy to maintain, and it will last for generations.

Glass Cookware: Glassware such as Pyrex or Corning Ware does not interact with the food chemically and may be used in the safe preparation of foods. Glass jars, bowls, and bottles are also better for storage than plastic, which reacts with the food or drink that is stored in it. Glass cookware is best for cooking liquid foods and steaming vegetables. It tends to heat unevenly and is not recommended for cooking foods that require precise temperature control. Foods tend to burn easily on the bottom of pots made of glass.

Cast-Iron Cookware: Cast-iron cookware is recommended for cooking because the iron entering the food benefits the system. Cast iron maintains heat well and diffuses it evenly, but it is slow to heat up and cool down and can react with acidic or alkaline foods. Cast iron requires seasoning before being used for the first time, and the oil-seasoned surface must be maintained, or it will rust.

Wok: The Chinese wok, if made of stainless steel or iron, is a very useful, safe, and healthful cooking utensil. It is good for cooking foods lightly and quickly to maintain food enzyme value.

Parchment Paper: Parchment paper combines the best qualities of covered baking and steaming. The parchment paper seals in moisture and, as the ingredients within cook, all the flavors are melded and preserved. Anything can be cooked in parchment. Meat, fish, shellfish, vegetables, and fruits are delicious when baked or steamed in tidy parchment packages that in French cuisine are known as *papillotes*. Meats and fish can be wrapped on a generous base of seasoned aromatics such as vegetables and herbs. The papillotes can be assembled up to 5 hours ahead and refrigerated until ready to use. Simple folded papillotes can be cut open and placed on each plate to create a unique presentation. Parchment paper is also reusable.

STRUCTURING YOUR DIET

We all need to establish our own optimum diets. Climate, activity, and metabolism all affect individual dietary needs. The main elements of structuring an optimum diet can be broken down into two food groups: cleansers and builders. Fruits, vegetables, and herbs are the body's cleansers. They are invaluable for mobilizing toxins and facilitating their elimination. Fruits, vegetables, and herbs keep the body clean and light. The body builders are comprised mainly of protein foods such as meats, dairy products, whole grains, avocados, mushrooms, tofu, beans, nuts, and seeds. An unbalanced ratio of these foods congests the body because they are mucus forming and overly acidic. This is true particularly for meats and dairy products. Other "congestors" are breads, cakes, cookies, candies, soft drinks, sugar products, flour, noodles, potatoes, corn, and all processed chemical foods. Eating too much congesting food can block the body functions and lead to stagnation and illness. Foods such as cold-pressed oils and organic butter act as "lubricators," as well as nourishers, which aid the mucous membranes, joints, tendons, ligaments, and elimination. Only a little of the lubricating and congesting food is required. Chemicals in the diet and overeating both stress the liver, digestive system, heart, kidneys, blood, and brain. *Diet increases stress, or reduces it. It can create disease, or help heal illness.*

It is important to remember that enzymes in raw food aid in the digestive process, and this takes the stress off having to borrow them from the body's enzyme reserve. Eating mostly raw food takes the stress off the endocrine system and preserves the lipase needed for proper metabolism of vitamins, minerals, and fats.

The foods we eat have a role in changing the body's size, shape, sexual responsiveness, and mental acuity. Read the labels of commercialized products before buying them. As we become aware and understand the nature of food, and learn how to create a healthful impact by making informed, intelligent choices, we begin to heal ourselves, our families and friends, and our earthly home.

EARTH PRAYER

The quality of our present and future lives can be willed now. It is essential to acknowledge and respect our deep connection with Nature. Let us work for and toward "The spirit of Truth" (one of all and for all). We open ourselves to learning when we summon the courage to change and leave arrogance, ignorance, greed, self-delusions, and vanities behind. When we are compelled toward this sacred doorway, the advancing motion of evolution is enhanced through harmony, change, enlightenment, and spiritual restoration.

—Carrie L'Esperance

NOTES

INTRODUCTION

1. Edgar Cayce Readings 288-038, quoted in Harold J. Reilly & Ruth Hagy Brod, *The Edgar Cayce Handbook for Health Through Drugless Therapy* (New York: Macmillan, 1975).
2. Bill Mollison, *Permaculture* (Tyalgum, Australia: Tagari Publications, 1988 and 1992).
3. Sogyal Rinpoche, *The Tibetan Book of Living and Dying* (New York: Harper Collins, 1992).

CHAPTER 1

1. Clarissa Pinkola Estés, *Women Who Run with the Wolves* (New York: Ballantine Books, 1992).
2. Dr. N.W. Walker, *Raw Vegetable Juices* (New York: The Berkeley Publishing Group, 1987).
3. George Ohsawa, *You Are All Sanpaku* (Secaucus, NJ: Citadel Press, 1965).
4. Edgar Cayce Readings 5439-1, quoted in *The Edgar Cayce Handbook for Health Through Drugless Therapy.*
5. Dr. Bernard Jensen, *Tissue Cleansing Through Bowel Management* (Escondido, CA: Bernard Jensen, 1981).

CHAPTER 2

1. Ilza Veith, *Nei Ching: The Yellow Emperor's Classic of Internal Medicine* (Berkeley, CA: University of California, 1972).
2. Dr. Elson Haas, MD, *Staying Healthy with the Seasons* (Berkeley, CA: Celestial Arts, 1981).
3. Vicki Noble, *Shakti Woman* (New York: Harper Collins, 1991).

CHAPTER 3

1. James Redfield, *The Celestine Prophecy* (New York: Warner Books, 1993).
2. Fannie Merritt Farmer, *The Boston Cooking School Cookbook* (Boston: Little Brown & Co., 1959).
3. Harold J. Reilly & Ruth Hagy Brod, *The Edgar Cayce Handbook for Health Through Drugless Therapy.*
4. Dr. Elson Haas, *Staying Healthy with the Seasons.*
5. Louise Tenney, *Today's Healthy Eating* (Provo, UT: Woodland Books, 1986).
6. Metabolic regulation means all physical and chemical changes within the body involving energy and material transformations.
7. Harold J. Reilly & Ruth Hagy Brod, *The Edgar Cayce Handbook for Health Through Drugless Therapy.*
8. Burt Green, *The Grains Cookbook* (New York: Workman Publishing, 1988).
9. Stanley Burroughs, *The Master Cleanser* (Kailua, HI: Stanley Burroughs, 1976).

CHAPTER 4

1. Eliot Cowan, *Plant Spirit Medicine* (Mill Spring, NC: Swan Raven & Co., 1995).
2. Minute vascular processes on the free surface of a membrane.
3. Ilza Veith, *Nei Ching: The Yellow Emperor's Classic of Internal Medicine.*
4. Harold J. Reilly & Ruth Hagy Brod, *The Edgar Cayce Handbook for Health Through Drugless Therapy.*
5. Dr. Henry Bieler, *Food Is Your Best Medicine* (New York: Ballantine Books, 1965).
6. William LeSassier, quoted in *Staying Healthy with the Seasons.*
7. Nathan Pritikin, Leonard J. Hofer, *Live Longer Now* (New York: Grosset & Dunlop, 1974).
8. Stanley Burroughs, *Healing for the Age of Enlightenment,* quoted in *Staying Healthy with the Seasons.*
9. Dr. Henry Bieler, *Food Is Your Best Medicine.*

10. Elson Haas, *Staying Healthy with the Seasons.*
11. Edgar Cayce Readings 1657-002, quoted in *The Edgar Cayce Handbook for Health Through Drugless Therapy.*
12. Albert Einstein, *The World as I See It,* trans. Allan Harris (Secaucus, NJ: Citadel Press, 1979).
13. Louise Tenney, *Today's Healthy Eating.*
14. Elson Haas, *Staying Healthy with the Seasons.*
15. Hannah Kroeger, *Good Health Through Special Diets* (Boulder, CO: Hannah Kroeger, 1971).
16. Peter Blue Cloud, *Clans of Many Nations* (Fredonia, NY: White Pine Press, 1995).

CHAPTER 5

1. Cazekiel, quoted in James Gilliland, *Becoming Gods* (Spring Mill, NC: Wildflower Press, 1996).
2. Adelle G. Dawson, *Herbs, Partners in Life* (Rochester, VT: Healing Arts Press, 1991).
3. Hannah Kroeger, *Good Health Through Special Diets.*
4. Dr. Bernard Jensen, *Tissue Cleansing Through Bowel Management.*

CHAPTER 6

1. Alberto Villoldo and Erik Jendresen, *Island of the Sun* (Rochester, VT: Destiny Books, 1992).
2. Tom Brown, *Tom Brown's Guide to Wild Edibles and Medicinal Plants* (New York: Berkeley Books, 1985).
3. Lavon J. Dunne, *Nutrition Almanac* third edition (New York: McGraw-Hill, 1990).
4. Jack London, *The Call of the Wild and White Fang* (New York: Bantam Books, 1981).

CHAPTER 7

1. Dr. Bernard Jensen, *Tissue Cleansing Through Bowel Management.*
2. Dr. K.M. Nadkarni, *Indian Materia Medica* vol. 1 & 2 (Bombay: Popular Prakashan Private LTD, 1976).
3. Edgar Cayce Readings 440-2, quoted in *The Edgar Cayce Handbook for Health Through Drugless Therapy.*
4. Hannah Kroeger, *Good Health Through Special Diets.*
5. Dr. Bernard Jensen, *Tissue Cleansing Through Bowel Management*
6. Claire Nahmiad, *Earth Magic* (Rochester, VT: Destiny Books, 1994).
7. Maria Trebin, *Health from God's Garden* (Rochester, VT: Healing Arts Press, 1986).
8. Claire Nahmiad, *Earth Magic* (London: Octopus Books, 1980).
9. Arabella Boxer and Philippa Back, *The Herb Book.*
10. Edgar Cayce Readings 1688-7 and 257-254, quoted in *The Edgar Cayce Handbook for Health Through Drugless Therapy.*

CHAPTER 8

1. Eliot Cowan, *Plant Spirit Medicine.*
2. Arabella Boxer and Philippa Back, *The Herb Book.*
3. Frank W. Gunther, *Kombucha* (Naples, FL: Valentine Communication Corp., 1994).
4. Ibid.
5. Ibid.

CHAPTER 9

1. Edgar Cayce Readings 2981-3, quoted in *The Edgar Cayce Handbook for Health Through Drugless Therapy.*
2. Harold J. Reilly & Ruth Hagy Brod, *The Edgar Cayce Handbook for Health Through Drugless Therapy.*
3. Herman Aihar, *Acid and Alkaline* (Oroville, CA: George Ohsawa Macrobiotic Foundation, 1986).

SELECTED BIBLIOGRAPHY

Aihar, Herman, *Acid and Alkaline* (Oroville, CA: George Ohsawa Macrobiotic Foundation, 1986).

Argüelles, José, *The Mayan Factor: Path Beyond Technology* (Santa Fe, NM: Bear & Co., 1987).

Bieler, Henry, M.D., *Food Is Your Best Medicine* (New York: Ballantine Books, 1965).

Blum, Jeanne, *Woman Heal Thyself* (Boston: Charles E. Tuttle Co., Inc., 1995).

Boxer, Arabella, and Philippa Back, *The Herb Book* (London: Octopus Books, 1980).

Brown, Tom, *Tom Brown's Guide to Wild Edibles and Medicinal Plants* (New York: Berkeley Books, 1985).

Burroughs, Stanley, *The Master Cleanser* (Kailua, HI: Stanley Burroughs, 1971).

Chisti, Hakim, N.D., *The Traditional Healer's Handbook* (Rochester, VT: Healing Arts Press, an imprint of Inner Traditions International, 1988 and 1991).

Cloud, Peter Blue, *Clans of Many Nations* (Fredonia, NY: White Pine Press, 1995).

Cowan, Eliot, *Plant Spirit Medicine* (Mill Spring, NC: Swan Raven & Co., 1995).

Davis, Adele, *Let's Get Well* (Bergenfield, NJ: The New American Library, 1965).

Dawson, Adele, *Herbs, Partners in Life* (Rochester, VT: Healing Arts Press, 1991).

Dunne, Lavon J., *Nutrition Almanac,* third edition (New York: McGraw-Hill, 1990).

Einstein, Albert, *The World As I See It*, trans. Allan Harris (Secaucus, NJ: Citadel Press, 1979).

Emerson, Ralph Waldo, *Essays: First and Second Series* (New York: Vintage Books, 1990).

Estés, Clarissa Pinkola, *Women Who Run with the Wolves* (New York: Ballantine Books, 1992).

Farmer, Fannie Merritt, *The Boston Cooking School Cookbook* (Boston: Little Brown & Co., 1959).

Gilliland, James, *Becoming Gods* (Mill Spring, NC: Wildflower Press, 1996).

Green, Burt, *The Grains Cookbook* (New York: Workman Publishing, 1988).

Gunther, Frank W., *Kombucha* (Naples, FL: Valentine Communication Corp., 1994).

Haas, Elson, M.D., *Staying Healthy with the Seasons* (Berkeley, CA: Celestial Arts, 1981).

Hakim, Shaykh, and Chishti Moinuddin, *The Book of Sufi Healing* (New York: Inner Traditions, 1985).

Heline, Corinne, *Color and Music in the New Age* (Marina Del Rey, CA: DeVorsee & Co., 1982).

Jarvis, D. C., M.D., *Folk Medicine* (New York: Henry Holt & Co., 1958).

Jensen, Dr. Bernard, *Tissue Cleansing Through Bowel Management* (Escondido, CA: Bernard Jensen, 1981).

Katzen, Mollie, *Moosewood Cookbook* (Berkeley, CA: Ten Speed Press, 1977).

Kroeger, Hannah, *Good Health Through Special Diets* (Boulder, CO: Hannah Kroeger, 1971).

Madison, Deborah with Edward Brown, *The Greens Cookbook* (New York: Bantam Books, 1987).

Mollison, Bill, *Permaculture* (Tyalgum, Australia: Tagari Publications, 1988 and 1992).

Morningstar, Amadea, *The Ayurveda Cookbook* (Santa Fe, NM: Lotus Press, 1990).

Nahmiad, Claire, *Earth Magic* (Rochester, VT: Destiny Books, an imprint of Inner Traditions International, 1994).

Noble, Vicki, *Shakti Woman* (New York: Harper Collins, 1991).

Ohsawa, George, *You Are All Sanpaku* (Secaucus, NJ: Citadel Press, 1965).

Redfield, James, *The Celestine Prophecy* (New York: Warner Books, Inc., 1993).

Reilly, Harold J., and Ruth Hagy Brod, *The Edgar Cayce Handbook for Health Through Drugless Therapy* (New York: Macmillan, 1975).

Rodale, J., and Staff, *The Prevention Method for Better Health* (London: Rodale Press, 1960).

Santillo, Humbart, *Food Enzymes: The Missing Link to Radiant Health* (Prescott, AZ: Hohm Press, 1987).

Sogyal, Rinpoche, *The Tibetan Book of Living and Dying* (New York: Harper Collins, 1992).

Tenney, Louise, *Today's Healthy Eating* (Provo, UT: Woodland Books, 1986).

Tisserand, Robert, *The Art of Aromatherapy* (Rochester, VT: Healing Arts Press, 1977).

Trebin, Maria, *Health from God's Garden* (Rochester, VT: Healing Arts Press, 1986).

Villoldo, Alberto, and Erik Jendresen, *Island of the Sun* (Rochester, VT: Destiny Books, an imprint of Inner Traditions, 1992).

Walker, N. W., M.D., *Raw Vegetable Juices* (New York: The Berkeley Publishing Group, 1987).

Weinberger, Stanley, *Parasites: An Epidemic in Disguise* (Larkspur, CA: Healing Within Products, 1993).

Weiner, Michael, *Earth Medicine, Earth Food* (New York: Ballantine Books, 1980).

SOURCES

AEG Juicer, 7811 Montrose Road, Potomac, MD 20874, 1-800-705-5559.

The American Association of Naturopathic Physicians, 2366 Eastlake Avenue E., Suite 322, Seattle, WA 98102. Write for brochures and referral information; cost $5.00.

The American Herbalists Guild, P.O. Box 746555, Arvada, CO 80006, (303) 423-8800.

Herbs for Life, P.O. Box 40028, Sarasota, FL 34278, (941) 362-9255.

CERTIFIERS OF WATER FILTERS

National Sanitation Foundation, 4151 Naperville Road, Ann Arbor, MI 48106, (708) 505-0160.

David Diagnostics, Inc., 46-01 Broadway, Astoria, NY 11103, (718) 278-7676.

Water Quality Association, 3475 Plymouth Road, P.O. Box 1468, Lisle, IL 60532, (313) 769-8010.

Nitrite test strips for screening well water for nitrite contamination.
Suburban Water Testing Laboratories, 4600 Kutztown Road, Temple, PA 19560, 1-800-433-6595 or (215) 929-3666. Offers a complete line of water-testing services. Kits shipped with sampling instructions.

Ozark Water Service and Analytical Lab, 114 Spring Street, Sulphur Springs, AR 72768. For water consultations, call free, 1-800-835-8908.

MAIL-ORDER ORGANIC WINE SOURCES

Chartrand Imports, P.O. Box 1319, Rockland, ME 04841, (207) 594-7300. Organic wines available nationwide.

Frey Vineyards, 14000 Tomki Road, Redwood Valley, CA 95470, (707) 485-5177. Mail-order distributor for French and California organic wines.

The Organic Wine Company, 1592 Union Street, San Francisco, CA 94123, 1-888-ECO-WINE.

Fetzer, Valley Oaks, 13601 East Side Road, P.O. Box 611, Hopland, CA 95449, (707) 744-1250 Sells certified organic French wines in the western U.S.

MISCELLANEOUS

Yellowwood, The Ancient Cookfire Retreat. For information write the author through Healing Arts Press, One Park Street, Rochester, VT 05767

Dr. Parcells System of Scientific Living, Inc., 1605 Coal Avenue S.E., Albuquerque, NM 87106, (505) 247-2744.

Herbal Handbook for Farm and Stable (Levy) and *Keep Your Pet Healthy the Natural Way* (Lazarus), The Penn Herb Company, 1-800-523-9971.

To order Kombucha tea culture by mail: Gem Cultures, 30301 Sherwood Road, Fort Bragg, CA 95437, (707) 964-2922. Recommended reading: *Kombucha* by Gunther W. Frank and others available through Valentine Communication Corporation, P.O. Box 11089, Naples, FL 33941, 1-800-321-0416.

There are many good flaxseed oils on the market. A pure, high-quality hempseed oil is available through The Ohio Hempery Incorporated, 7002 S.R. 329, Guysville, Ohio 45735, 1-800-BUY-HEMP.

Penn Herb Co., 10601 Decatur Road, Philadelphia, PA 19154, 1-800-523-9971. Mail-order herbs and vegicaps.

Crystal Star Herbal Nutrition, 20065-B Highway 108, Sonora, CA 95370. For cleansing and fasting tea.

Pinkroot is available through the Penn Herb Co., 10601 Decatur Road, Philadelphia, PA 19154, 1-800-523-9971.

Dr. John Christopher, The Herb Shop, P.O. Box 77, Springville, UT 84663, 1-800-453-1406 or -1969. Herbs and VF Liquid herbal formulas. "BF&C" formula for skin trouble. "CSK" Plus for weight control. "AR-1" for arthritis. "FEN-LB" builds and strengthens the small and large intestines. "Adrenetone" to rebuild adrenals. "Juni-Pars" for the kidneys and bladder. "Prospallate" for kidney stones.

Herb Research Foundation's Hotline can provide reliable information about benefits, dose, and safety for more than 200 herbs. (303) 449-2265.

Dr. Bernard Jensen, 243 Old Wagon Road, Escondido, CA 92027, (760) 749-2727. To obtain *Tissue Cleansing Through Bowel Management*.

Edgar Cayce Foundation, P.O. Box 595, Virginia Beach, VA 23451-0595, (804) 428-3588. For further research into the readings of Edgar Cayce.

Burroughs Books, 8905 Crater Hill Road, Newcastle, CA 95658. Write for a list of books including *The Master Cleanser*.

INDEX OF SYMPTOMS
AND ILLNESSES

INDEX OF PLANTS AND HERBS
(AND DERIVATIVES)

ABOUT THE AUTHOR

Carrie L'Esperance has studied many healing systems from the world's various cultures—past and present—for more than twenty-five years. She has blended her research and the practical application of the principles studied into one dynamic system, which is the basis for her book *The Seasonal Detox Diet.*

Carrie is a certified iridologist and develops health programs for individuals using eye analysis to indicate their nutritional requirements. Healthy circulation of the body's six systems of detoxification, and tissue cleansing for vitality and longevity, are integrated into her programs as preventive health measures. Carrie has been perfecting the art of fasting on herself for more than fifteen years and has had successful results for both her and her clients.

Carrie is the founding director of Women for Wellness, which was established in 1985 in the San Francisco Bay area. This not-for-profit organization is dedicated to the wellness of humanity and to planetary transformation. Developing recycling programs, planting trees, urban gardening for charity, and alternative health education are some of the various projects implemented by this organization.

Carrie's professional experience in the culinary arts began in 1981 with her work in the innovative food world of San Francisco. Six years working for gourmet establishments such as The Oakville Grocery, Neiman Marcus, and California Sunshine Caviar Company enriched her experience in the preparation and service of fine foods and wines.

Throughout her adult life, Carrie has had an active career in the creative arts, including more than 20 years of professional dance training and yoga, and she currently does freelance work in the commercial film industry as a photo stylist. She has also received numerous awards for her paintings and photographs.

As for her future plans, Carrie says, "I love the land and nature. My dream is to work with the land and develop the Yellowwood Retreat based on permaculture design. Carrie currently lives in San Francisco, California.

BOOKS OF RELATED INTEREST

TRADITIONAL FOODS ARE YOUR BEST MEDICINE
Improving Health and Longevity with Native Nutrition
by Ronald F. Schmid, N.D.

FOOD ALLERGIES AND FOOD INTOLERANCE
The Complete Guide to Their Identification and Treament
by Jonathan Brostoff, M.D., and Linda Gamlin

MEALS THAT HEAL
A Nutraceutical Approach to Diet and Health
by Lisa Turner

WHOLE FOOD BIBLE
How to Select and Prepare Safe, Healthful Foods
by Chris Kilham

FOOD COMBINING FOR HEALTH
Get Fit with Foods that Don't Fight
by Doris Grant and Jean Joice

AYURVEDIC HEALING CUISINE
By Harish Johari

THE CLAY CURE
Natural Healing from the Earth
by Ran Knishinsky

GENETICALLY ENGINEERED FOOD: CHANGING THE NATURE OF NATURE
What You Need to Know to Protect Yourself, Your Family, and Our Planet
by Martin Teitel, Ph.D., and Kimberly A. Wilson

Inner Traditions • Bear & Company
P.O. Box 388
Rochester, VT 05767
1-800-246-8648
www.InnerTraditions.com

Or contact your local bookseller